FIT AND HEALTHY
AT 40+

GW00493919

FIT AND HEALTHY AT 40+

JUDY BYRNE

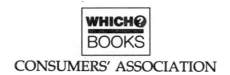

CONSUMERS' ASSOCIATION

Which? Books are commissioned and researched by
The Association for Consumer Research and published by
Consumers' Association, 2 Marylebone Road, NW1 4DF

Distributed by the Penguin Group;
Penguin Books Ltd, 27 Wrights Lane, London W8 5TZ

First edition June 1994

British Library Cataloguing in Publication Data

Byrne, Judy
('Which?' Consumer Guides)
I. Title   II. Series
613.0434
ISBN 0 85202 555 6

Cover photographs by courtesy of ACE/Mugshots, ACE/Bill
Bachmann and John Walmsley

Typeset by Tech-Set, Gateshead, Tyne and Wear
Printed and bound by Firmin-Didot (France), 27018
Groupe Herissey

CONTENTS

INTRODUCTION   7

QUIZ   10

1 WHY EXERCISE?   11

2 WHICH EXERCISE?   37

3 HEALTHY EATING   65

4 SMOKING AND DRINKING   91

5 TIME OF CHANGE   113

6 KEEPING HEALTH PROBLEMS AT BAY   137

7 GOOD STRESS GUIDE   165

8 LOOKING FORWARD   201

ANSWERS TO QUIZ   212

USEFUL ADDRESSES   215

RECOMMENDED READING   219

INDEX   221

INTRODUCTION

AGEING begins at birth. Most of us disregard it or pretend nothing is changing for us until somewhere around the 40 mark. Then we may start worrying about what ageing is, what might be happening to us and whether there is anything we can do to slow it down.

One aim of this book is to answer some of these questions we tend to start asking ourselves around the middle years of our lives – questions such as 'Is there anything we can do to maximise the number of years we have to look forward to?' and, perhaps even more pertinently, 'Is there anything we can do to improve the quality of those years?'

The bad news is that current research suggests we are not on the brink of finding the secret of eternal youth. Some of the cells in our bodies – for example, skin and blood cells – start off looking as though they will carry on growing and renewing themselves until the end of time. As the years pass, however, the cell-renewal process gradually wears out: the process itself slows down, and the replacement cells are not 'as good as new', as a comparison of a 20-year-old and a 60-year-old skin will show. Other cells, such as those in the kidney, brain, heart muscle and the lens of the eye, don't renew themselves at all. Once they wear out, the body cannot replace them, even if medical technology increasingly can via transplants.

But it now seems that some of our cells, such as those that form the fibrous skeleton of our connective tissue, come programmed to reproduce themselves only a limited number of times. Even when such cells are frozen for years and thawed, they seem to retain the memory of how many times they have already divided and how many more they have left.

Hoping that scientists will announce the ultimate breakthrough in time for us is, on present knowledge, not looking like an optimum strategy.

But there is good news too, and plenty of it also comes from the research front. Even those of us on the 'wrong' side of the 40 mark will find that exercise will make us significantly fitter, and have spin-off benefits ranging from making us feel more relaxed and cheerful to helping us sleep better. Exercising regularly, along with eating healthily, can also decrease the likelihood that we will be victims of the major killers in our society: coronary heart disease and cancer. Giving up smoking, whatever age we are, improves our health, fitness – and future prospects – enormously.

How much it matters to each of us whether we are as fit and healthy as we possibly can be is very much a personal decision. That also goes for what we are prepared to change about our present life styles in order to achieve our goals. This book does not lay down rules for being fit and healthy at 40-plus. It does aim to spell out the facts we need to know to make those choices informed ones. And it is packed with strategies and tips for making us fitter and healthier in mind and body with minimum effort and maximum effect.

Another aim of this book is to redress a historic imbalance in Western society, by putting as much emphasis on mental as on physical health. We are only beginning to realise the complexity of mind–body relationships, and to understand some of the ways in which our thinking processes influence how healthy we are and feel. Our ability to deal sensibly, even creatively, with stress, along with our attitude to ourselves and the opportunities available to us, is as important as our blood pressure and fitness in shaping the quality of the future we have in front of us.

The first three chapters – 'Why Exercise?', 'Which Exercise?' and 'Healthy Eating' – explain how beneficial exercise and diet can be. These chapters also describe how exercise and diet can most easily and effectively be incorporated into our life styles with a minimum of disruption and a maximum pay-off – and with an emphasis on enjoyment.

Chapter 4, 'Smoking and Drinking', discusses the effects of alcohol, caffeine and nicotine on our health. It spells out how the risks of continuing to smoke increase with every decade and how giving up, even late in life, improves health prospects enormously. It gives practical advice on how to stop smoking, and it contains good news for you if you like to have a drink or two.

Chapter 5, 'Time of Change', looks at the major physical changes that occur in men and in women from around 40 onwards and the pluses and problems of love in middle age and beyond, and discusses the implications surrounding the decision by some women to opt for late motherhood. It helps women confronting the menopause answer the question: 'Is hormone replacement therapy for me?'

Chapter 6, 'Keeping Health Problems at Bay', considers some of the health problems that become more likely after the 40 mark, and how best to prevent or cope with them. Chapter 7, 'Good Stress Guide', considers how sources of stress can differ at different stages of our lives and gives successful strategies for dealing with both overstress and its mirror image, understress.

The final chapter, 'Looking Forward', looks at the psychological challenge of being 40-plus and at the new opportunities that can open up for us in the second half of our lives. So much depends on our approach. The middle years can be a time when we go into mourning for our lost youth and opportunities and for all we now know we will never do. Or it can be second-chance time, when many of us find ourselves with more time and possibly more money, often post-child-rearing, to concentrate on ourselves and discover and meet our own needs.

We know we'll never now captain the England test team at cricket or set a new world record for the women's 100 metres, but our best years are not necessarily behind us. They may well be ahead. This chapter discusses how we can use goal planning to help us ensure that we are less haphazard about what we achieve in the second half of our lives than we may have been in the first.

Throughout this book, when organisations are mentioned and marked with an asterisk (*) you will find fuller details listed under Useful Addresses on pp. 215–7. There is fuller information about books that are marked in the text with a double asterisk (**) in the list of Recommended Reading on pp. 219–20. In both lists, details are given chapter by chapter, and in the order in which a book or organisation is first mentioned in the text.

FIT AND HEALTHY AT 40+ QUIZ

Questions:

1. There are established links between diet and which of the following illnesses: (a) heart disease (b) cancer of the uterus (c) cancer of the gall bladder (d) cancer of the colon (e) prostate cancer (f) breast cancer (g) osteoporosis (h) stroke

2. Fitness inevitably decreases with age. Is this (a) true or (b) false?

3. Who was older: (a) Winston Churchill when he first became Prime Minister, or (b) Mary Wesley when she published her first novel?

4. Being overweight is a bigger health hazard if most of the excess is around the waist than if we wear it around the hips. Is this: (a) true or (b) false?

5. What proportion of smokers are reckoned to die of smoking-related diseases: (a) one in 40 (b) one in 20 (c) one in 12 (d) one in 7 or (e) one in 3?

6. Are commercial diet foods more likely to help you lose more: (a) lbs or (b) £££s?

7. How much can passive smoking increase your risk of lung cancer: (a) not at all (b) to twice as much (c) to three times as much?

8. What proportion of women over the age of 70 can expect to have a hip fracture within a five-year period? (a) 1 in 10 (b) 1 in 6 (c) 1 in 4 (d) 1 in 2 or (e) 2 in 3?

9. What percentage of illnesses reported to GPs are believed to be stress-related: (a) 90 (b) 75 (c) 50 (d) 35 (e) 20 or (f) 10?

For the answers, see pp.212–13.

CHAPTER 1

WHY EXERCISE?

EVEN in the earliest months of life, before the nervous system is fully wired up, before the body has reached a fraction of its maximum size or its reproductive potential, it has begun to age physically. However, it is not until around 25 to 30 that ageing begins to be equated with the beginnings of physical decline rather than physical development or maturation.

On average, bones start to reduce in size and weight in the mid-30s, and muscle power also slowly declines from about 40 onwards. The heart becomes less powerful and every year loses a percentage of its ability to push the blood around the body. Between 30 and 50, blood vessels become about a third narrower, on average. Muscle fibre disappears at the rate of a few per cent every 10 years. By 65, we burn up about 5 per cent fewer calories than we did at 25, so if we continue to eat the same amount of food, the excess turns to fat.

In the face of this grim and seemingly relentless decline, medical research is now beginning to examine to what extent these average rates of physical decline are the result of simple disuse rather than inevitable deterioration. And the evidence for the former is encouraging. It comes from two different sources: studies in which people, including some in their 90s, were put on exercise programmes and made quite astounding improvements in their fitness, and surveys where the fitness levels of people of different ages were assessed to see whether these related to their age or how active they were.

The results boil down to the same conclusion – 'use it or lose it'. Fitness does not have to be related to the number of birthdays we have clocked up. We can choose to improve it, however long we have been walking (or not walking much) around planet Earth.

Does fitness matter?

Whether you concern yourself with how fit you are is, of course, a personal choice. Sadly, it is one many people never really make. They drift into unfitness by default, without considering what the long-term consequences of their inactivity might be, and often without any accurate idea how unfit or inactive they really are. There is now convincing scientific evidence that the more active you are, the less likely you are to suffer heart disease and other major Western-world killer diseases. Being fit not only lengthens the odds on the quantity of life you can expect, but will also almost certainly improve the quality. That message is apparently yet to be widely acted upon in Britain.

The National Fitness Survey for the Sports Council and the Health Education Authority studied a random sample of 6000 people between February and November 1990, and was the most comprehensive ever carried out in England. The survey report, *Activity and Fitness Matters*, revealed that 80 per cent of people believe they are fit – and most of them are kidding themselves.

For example, a third of the men tested and two-thirds of the women couldn't walk for long at a reasonable pace (about three miles an hour) up a 1-in-20 slope. After several minutes, they became breathless and had to slow down or stop. About half the women aged 55 and over tested found that walking even on flat ground at that pace for several minutes proved to be severe exertion. In addition, nearly a third of the men and half of the women from 65 to 74 did not have enough strength in their thigh muscles to get out of a chair without using their arms to help them. Half the women 55 and over could not climb stairs without using a hand-rail for help.

Eighty-one per cent of men between 45 and 54 fell below the target level of fitness for their age group – which was particularly worrying given the high risk for this group of coronary heart disease from other factors.

The survey (which was sponsored by Allied Dunbar) found that people are as unrealistic in their self-assessment of how active they really are as they are about their own fitness. Around six out of ten men and seven out of ten women in the lowest activity level (those who had not had even a 20-minute burst of a mixture of moderate and vigorous activity *once* in the previous four weeks) described themselves as very or fairly fit. Nearly half the men in that least-active group and nearly two-thirds of the women also believed they were either very or fairly active. But, apart from the fact that they are unrealistic about their fitness levels, are these people really missing out?

The anti-exercise lobby loves to cite the case of Jim Fixx, America's leading jogging guru, who dropped dead running in 1984. That, they claimed, settled the argument against exercise once and for all. But Fixx had been extremely overweight, had had high cholesterol levels for many years and as a young man had smoked heavily. He also had a family history of serious heart disease.

In addition, a sample of one never did prove anything – whether the example cited is Fixx or the legendary, sedentary 90-year-old smoker and drinker who has never had a day's illness in his or her life and whom the anti-exercisers love to point out as living proof that an unhealthy life style never did hurt anybody. Some individuals are lucky enough to be genetically predisposed to withstand abuse that would kill the rest of us decades sooner. Finding out by trial and error if you are one of them, however, is a bit like playing Russian roulette.

Set against that tale of one unfortunate man and enduring myths of survival against the odds is the evidence collected by a team led by Professor Jerry Morris, one of the earliest pioneers of research into the protection that exercise gives us against death from heart disease. Professor Morris discovered more than 30 years ago that bus conductors, who had a more active working day climbing up and down bus stairs collecting fares than drivers did, also had fewer heart attacks than the drivers. Since 1976, he and his colleagues have been monitoring the physical activities and the health of 10,000 civil servants. In 1990, they reported that 272 men in the study had by then died of coronary heart disease and 202 had developed non-fatal heart disease. They found that men who took part in vigorous sports – such as swimming, tennis, football, hockey, hill climbing or rowing –

two or three times a week had only a third of the risk of heart disease of those who did not.

Fitness facts

Some of the most important benefits of regular physical activity – and these are backed by a wealth of scientific evidence – are that exercise

- lowers the chance of early death
- reduces the risk of coronary heart disease (which kills someone in the UK every three minutes)
- reduces the likelihood of strokes
- reduces blood cholesterol levels
- improves circulation
- can lower the blood pressure of people with hypertension (the early warning signal of possible problems such as strokes ahead)
- increases stamina
- can help prevent osteoporosis, the 'brittle bones' condition resulting from bone-mass loss that makes elderly women (and increasingly, as they live longer, elderly men) more prone to breaks
- makes and keeps muscles strong
- keeps joints flexible
- helps improve posture
- helps keep body-weight down, thus reducing the risk of obesity-related diseases (which include diabetes, high blood pressure, gout, hiatus hernia, gallstones, osteoarthritis and cancers of the uterus, gall bladder and breast)
- reduces the risk of developing adult diabetes and can help non-insulin-dependent diabetics better manage their condition
- aids rehabilitation after a heart attack
- relieves stress and enhances mood
- improves co-ordination.

Many people who take regular exercise also report that it:

- gives them more self-confidence
- makes them feel more in control of their lives
- helps them to like their bodies better
- aids sleep
- quickens recovery when ill health does strike.

Components of fitness

Activity promotes fitness and fitness has three separate components. One of them is **suppleness**, or flexibility – the ability to bend, stretch, twist and turn through a full range of movement. A second is **strength** – the force we can exert when we push, pull and lift. The third is **stamina**, endurance or aerobic fitness – the ability to keep on going. It enables us to walk long distances briskly or to run for a bus without getting out of breath and exhausted.

Aerobic means using oxygen. Aerobic fitness is the ability to use the oxygen from the air we breathe to free energy for our muscles. People who are not aerobically fit are unable to do this for any length of time. Muscle strength and joint flexibility are pre-requisites for the sort of vigorous exercise we need to increase stamina. With stamina training we become able to breathe more deeply. Our hearts pump oxygen round our bodies and our muscles use it more efficiently. The more supple we are, the less likely we are to be accidentally injured when we are exercising. Strength protects us from sprains and strains, and tends to improve our posture. Activities that build stamina are also the ones that give us protection against heart disease and strokes. Thus each component of fitness not only helps promote the others but also has benefits in our everyday lives.

People who are more active increase the odds that they will live longer and live better in more subtle ways. They are making it more likely that they will be able to keep their independence further into old age. For example, a major break of a bone, like that of a leg or a hip, can be the beginning of the end of being able to manage at home alone for an elderly person, no matter how fiercely he or she values that independence.

Flexibility is not just about being able to pass some performance test in the gym. It is about being able to change light bulbs and tie shoelaces and get in and out of a car with ease. We keep supple by moving our joints through their whole range of movement every day. If we don't, they begin to stiffen and the range of movement becomes more limited. Strength is not an abstract measurement of muscle power but the ability to get up the stairs easily, carry the shopping and take off stubborn bottle-tops. Muscles become and stay stronger longer when they are pushed against resistance. If they aren't used regularly, they become weaker. Posture suffers, too. And not having the aerobic fitness we need can become dangerous when we find it difficult to avoid vigorous activity – such as running for a bus or shovelling snow from a driveway.

Cross-training is the name given to an activity programme which includes a mixture of exercises in order to increase aerobic fitness and build endurance, flexibility and strength (see p.39), and it is the approach that experts in sports medicine recommend. Besides being a good, balanced, all-round approach to getting our bodies working better, cross-training also has the bonus of built-in variety.

The fitness path

If you are unfit and you decide to commit yourself to becoming and staying fit, what would it entail? And what results could you realistically expect? Studies in which people in their 50s, 60s and beyond have been put on fitness programmes have shown that they can improve their physical condition just as dramatically as younger people can.

In 1988, Dr William Evans and his team at Tufts University in Boston reported having found that men between 60 and 72 were able to increase their muscle mass by 15 per cent and their strength by 200 per cent with regular exercise and weight-training. Men and women between 86 and 96 did only slightly less well. So it is never too late to begin, and the less fit you are to start with, the more quickly you will notice results. An eight-year study at the Institute for Aerobics Research in Dallas, Texas, which ended in 1989, found that those who gained most from a 30 to 35 minute programme of brisk walking six or seven days a week were those who had been the most sedentary.

Even a little exercise is better than none, according to the interim findings of the British Regional Heart Study, which has been looking at the health of nearly 8000 middle-aged men living in 24 towns in Britain. Over 10 years, 128 of the men randomly selected to take part in the survey have had strokes. Analysis of their levels of physical activity before they became ill showed that those who had been taking no exercise at all were six times more likely to have a stroke than those who were taking vigorous exercise regularly.

Perhaps even more encouragingly, the survey found that men who did only a little regular exercise got some protection, compared with those who did none. Some physical activity such as walking and playing a sport or having some recreational activity once a week seems enough to reduce the risk for men of having a heart attack or stroke. (Although the study did not test it, this probably applies to women, too.)

A recent American study found a similar picture, as the chart below shows. The fittest people had the lowest death rate. But at the other end of the scale, those who did even a little regular exercise, while they had slightly poorer survival odds than the very fittest, still fared much better than those who had no regular activity at all.

EVEN A LITTLE SAVES LIVES

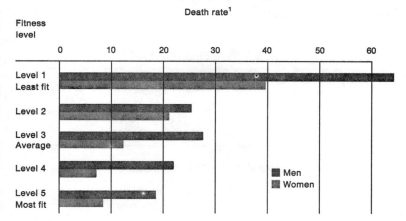

Source: Journal of the American Medical Association

In this trial, people who did nothing at all were two to three times more likely to die than people doing even a small amount of exercise. Death rate[1] here means the expected number of deaths for 1000 people over a period of 10 years, or 10,000 people over a year.

One common finding among all the studies is that the regular activity has to have been recent to have a beneficial effect. We have to keep it up to reap the rewards. Fitness slips away quite quickly once we stop; 10 weeks without regular activity and our fitness declines drastically. Exercise, it seems, has to be for life.

That fitness is related to the way we use our bodies, rather than how old we are, was confirmed by the National Fitness Survey. The survey found that some elderly people are as fit as or fitter than some men and women in their 20s, 30s and 40s. The average aerobic capacity of the fittest 10 per cent of men aged 65 to 74 was higher, it was discovered, than that of the least fit 10 per cent of men aged 25 to 34. The pattern for women was similar.

The report also found that the less active people were, the more likely they were either to have some condition that limited them in one or more of their everyday tasks, or to mention to interviewers that they suffered a chronic disease or injury, particularly heart disease, angina or breathlessness. The National Fitness Survey and the Health Survey for England, which was carried out the following year by the Office of Population, Censuses and Surveys for the Department of Health, used the same desirable activity levels for different age groups. They are shown in Tables 1 and 2, below:

Table 1: TARGET LEVELS SCALE

Age group (men and women)	Target activity level
16-34	Activity level 5
35-54	Activity level 4
55-74	Activity level 3

Table 2: ACTIVITY LEVELS SCALE

Level	Activity of 20 minutes' duration in the previous four weeks
Activity level 5	12 or more occasions of vigorous activity
Activity level 4	12 or more occasions of a mix of moderate and vigorous activity
Activity level 3	12 or more occasions of moderate activity
Activity level 2	5 to 11 occasions of a mix of moderate and vigorous activity
Activity level 1	1 to 4 occasions of a mix of moderate and vigorous activity
Activity level 0	None

Moderate covers activities such as long walks (two miles or more) at a brisk or fast pace; football, swimming, tennis, aerobics, cycling, table tennis, golf and social dancing – if they do not make you out of breath or sweaty; heavy DIY like mixing cement; heavy gardening such as digging; and heavy housework like spring cleaning. For exercise to be rated **vigorous**, you would have to become sweaty or out of breath. Vigorous exercises include hill-walking briskly; playing football, tennis or squash; running; or doing aerobics or cycling, or a job involving a great deal of climbing, lifting or carrying of heavy loads.

The National Fitness Survey found that the activity targets for their age levels were reached by fewer than one in five men and just over one in ten women between 45 and 54; by around one in three men and women between 55 and 64; and by only one in four men and one in five women between 65 and 74.

The importance of reaching these activity targets can be seen more clearly in the context of how the body functions.

Know your body

The **skeleton** is the framework that supports the body. It consists of more than 200 separate bones made of 67 per cent calcium salts and 33 per cent organic matter, mainly collagen. Some bones have a soft, fatty core, or marrow. The marrow's job is to produce new blood cells. Load-bearing exercise is a bone-builder and strengthener.

When two or more bones join together, they form a joint. Strong, flexible strips of tendon and ligament support the joints and hold them in place. Tendons attach muscle to the bone at a joint, and damage to a tendon is called a strain. Ligaments are attached to the bone either side of a joint and keep the bones together, both supporting them and allowing them to move at the same time. Damage to a ligament is a sprain.

Exercise can put stress on joints and can damage them if it is overdone or not done carefully enough, if the exercise is incorrect or inappropriate or is performed with insufficient warming up and stretching beforehand, or if it is done without the right equipment and the correct shoes (there are hints for choosing shoes in the next chapter). Footwear suitable for you and for what you are doing protects not only feet but also backs, legs and knees.

The knee, with two pieces of cartilage in the cavity, is the most vulnerable of joints. Cartilage is sensitive to wear and tear from strain during exercise. Knees actually suffer between one and three and one in four of all sports injuries, and a knee injury can have knock-on effects.

Varying the load on joint surfaces during exercise increases the flow of natural lubricant into the joint cavity and the flow of nutrients to the cartilage. This keeps friction between the moving parts to a minimum and protects the surfaces from damage. The right exercise done correctly strengthens the muscles, ligaments and tendons that support and protect joints, keeping them mobile and healthy and less likely to become stiff or even painful through the onset of joint conditions such as fibrositis, lumbago, sciatica and arthritis.

Muscle contraction causes all the movements our bodies make. We have around 650 muscles in all and they come in three varieties – smooth muscle, responsible for the automatic movements of internal organs such as our intestines; cardiac muscle, which drives the pump we call the heart; and the skeletal muscle, which is attached to bone and which is the muscle we use to make all our voluntary movements.

Muscles quickly lose strength with disuse, as you will know if you have ever seen a broken limb when the plaster cast is first taken off. Elderly women used to wearing firm corsets have found it exhausting to maintain posture without them for even half a day.

It used to be thought that an inevitable, steady fall-off of muscle power was linked with increasing age. We now know that there may be some small inevitable loss because some non-renewable nerve fibres die and a muscle is useless without its nerve. But much of what we thought was age-linked loss we now know is simply the result of underuse. And the decline from underuse is reversible.

Muscles always move bones by contracting or shortening themselves and pulling the bone with them, never by pushing bones around. When you bend your arm, for example, one muscle contracts and another lengthens, and when you want to straighten it again they reverse roles. Because muscle groups work in antagonistic pairs in this way, it is important not to over-develop some in training without corresponding attention to the complementary ones. For the same reason, it is an essential safety precaution to stretch muscles progressively when warming up before starting to exercise.

Muscles are made of tough, stringy tissues. If you were to cut a muscle and have a look at it in cross-section, you would find that it is actually a bundle of fibres. Each fibre in turn is composed of smaller fibrils, and each fibril consists of even smaller overlapping filaments of muscle protein. It is when protein filaments pull themselves over one another, ratchet-fashion, so that they overlap further, that muscles contract.

Repeated use of muscles improves their strength in two ways: more muscle cells become drawn into the activity, and the muscle cells make more contractile protein so each cell can generate more force. You can build up a considerable increase in strength over time without any increase in the overall size of the muscle. So don't let the prospect of bulging biceps put you off exercise.

The safe and effective approach to increasing muscle strength is repeatedly contracting muscles for about five seconds at a time. Holding contractions for too long produces a rise in blood pressure and heart rate which could go beyond what is healthy for you. But strengthened muscles help protect you against that potentially hazardous rise in blood pressure from, for example, having to lift or hold a heavy weight for a time while doing some DIY in the house or garden.

The **heart** is a blood-filled bag of muscle weighing around three-quarters of a pound in adults, and is about the size of a clenched fist. As in the case of other muscles, exercising it strengthens and enlarges it, enabling it to work more efficiently. Its job is to pump blood around the body through an extensive network of arteries, capillaries and veins, delivering nutrients to all the cells in the body and taking waste materials away.

At rest, the average heart beats between 70 and 80 times a minute, though it can be much lower in the very fit. Extremely fit athletes such as racing cyclists and Olympic swimmers often have pulses as low as 40. The heart pumps between one and five gallons of blood a minute depending on what the body needs at the time. The heart can pump blood a distance of about 60,000 miles a day. Every pound of excess fat we carry adds an extra 200 miles each day to the journey.

Like all the muscles of the body, the heart needs oxygen to work, and the harder it works the more oxygen it needs. It gets oxygen by pumping blood to the lungs to collect it. The oxygenated blood then returns to the heart to fuel it and then for distribution around the whole body. The veins carry the 'spent' blood, which has given up its oxygen and other nutrients and collected waste products and carbon dioxide, back to the heart to begin another cycle.

YOUR HEART AND HOW IT WORKS

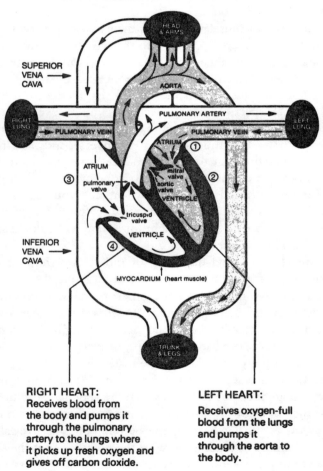

RIGHT HEART:
Receives blood from the body and pumps it through the pulmonary artery to the lungs where it picks up fresh oxygen and gives off carbon dioxide.

LEFT HEART:
Receives oxygen-full blood from the lungs and pumps it through the aorta to the body.

The more vigorously we exercise, the more our hearts speed up. The extent to which the heart is accelerated during exercise is important in determining how efficiently we are working towards becoming fitter, and is discussed in detail under Training zone, below. The speed with which the heartbeat returns to normal after strenuous exercise is an indicator of how fit we are.

The heart can keep doing its job efficiently only if it gets this constant supply of oxygenated and nutrient-rich blood via the coronary arteries, which branch off from the aorta (the main trunk artery). These arteries are no wider than a thin drinking straw and have a delicate lining which can become damaged and clogged. When the coronary arteries begin to become blocked by plaque – a condition that can be related to lack of exercise, high blood pressure or high blood cholesterol – the blood supply is affected. The first indication of this if we are lucky can be the sharp chest pains of angina, an early warning that generally responds to medication and life-style changes.

Exercise widens the arteries, so making it less likely that a blood clot will be able to block them completely. Exercise can also heal and remove plaque. Such blockages can cause thrombosis, heart attacks or strokes, depending on exactly where they occur.

Lungs are made up of about 750 million air sacs (or alveoli) which have a combined surface of about 60 square yards. We take in air through nose or mouth via the windpipe (or trachea) and into the lungs, which extract from it the oxygen we need and expel used air, which includes carbon dioxide. The air sacs are surrounded by a complex network of blood vessels, and it is in these that oxygen enters the bloodstream and waste carbon dioxide is extracted from it.

Below the lungs is the diaphragm, the wall of muscle at the bottom of the chest cavity which moves up and down and so controls the capacity of the lungs as we inhale and exhale. The intercostal muscles, the muscles between adjacent ribs, also move the ribs and increase the size of the cavity into which our lungs can expand when we breathe in. During exercise, we use neck muscles to increase the capacity of the lungs. During strenuous exercise, we should aim to get into a pattern of slow regular breathing – in through the nose, and out through the mouth, allowing the same time span (about two seconds) for each inhalation and each exhalation.

We breathe out not only gases but moisture as well. As our body temperature rises during vigorous exercise, so does the amount of moisture we expel – hence the need to take plenty of liquids during vigorous exercise. We need to have a little to drink at least once every 20 minutes. (But go easy on the quantity so you don't overload your stomach – a little often is best.) If we wait until we actually feel thirsty, we have left it later than is wise. Strenuous exercise can be tough enough, without simultaneously fighting the effects of mild dehydration as well.

In healthy people, training does not improve the lungs themselves, though if the respiratory muscles are weak they may become stronger. Usually the lungs and respiratory muscles do not limit our ability to exercise. Oxygen delivery to the muscles is determined by our circulation rather than our lungs, unless the lungs are actually diseased, as in emphysema. As we exercise, our circulation improves and our muscles become increasingly efficient at getting more oxygen from each drop of blood. Thus the more fit we become, the less easily we feel out of breath.

Metabolism is the chemical process by which the body turns food and oxygen into energy and warmth, leaving the excess to be stored as fat against future famine. We are fortunate in Western countries these days that famine is largely unknown. As we rarely turn to our fat stores to survive, we tend just to pile on the pounds with the passing years. (How to eat more healthily is covered in Chapter 3.) Exercise can improve muscle fitness, and that, in turn, will metabolise the food we eat more efficiently.

Fitness test

If you join a well-run gym or can afford to sign up with a personal trainer, the first thing that will be done is a test to find out how fit you are. But if you opt to get fit on your own, you should test yourself, both to ensure that you are working well within safe limits and so you can give yourself feedback about your progress. To check your pulse, you will need a stopwatch or a watch with a second-hand on it. Put your index and middle fingers where you can feel throbbing in the side of the neck (just below the jawline) or on the inside of the wrist. Count the beats for 15 seconds and multiply by four. (After strenuous exercise, the pulse rate of fit people drops speedily, so counting for a whole minute does not tell you what the rate was when you stopped exercising and started counting.)

You also need to know your resting pulse rate, which should be taken when you are really rested and relaxed, ideally first thing in the morning before you have had anything to eat or drink. You might want to make a note of your resting pulse rate on Table 3, below.

Once you know how to take your pulse, you will need a stair-case, ideally with a step of about eight inches. To practise, step up on to the first step with your right foot, and then step up with your left. Step down again in the same order. Time yourself so that the process takes you five seconds. Then step up with your left foot first and your right and then step down again. This should also take five seconds. Once you have that mastered, you are ready to start.

To test yourself:

- Step up and down as you did in the practice session, stepping up and down with the right foot followed by the left and then the left followed by the right, for three minutes.
- Take your pulse now and record it as your exercise pulse on the table below.
- Rest for one minute and take your pulse again. Enter it on the chart as your recovery rate.

Table 3: PULSE-RATE RECORD

	Example	Yours
Resting rate	80	
Exercise rate (during or after exercise)	135	
Recovery rate (a minute after exercise)	105	

The fitter you become the stronger your heart beats, so it pumps more blood with each beat. This means that as your fitness increases, your resting pulse becomes lower, as does your exercise rate after the same amount of work. The fitter you are, the more quickly your pulse returns to the resting rate after strenuous exercise. So you can expect to see your recovery rate moving closer to your resting rate.

Training zone

Your training zone is the range in which ideally you want to keep your pulse for maximum benefit while you are doing aerobic exercise. Let it go much higher and you could go beyond what you can safely ask of your heart. Let it stay lower and you are not working hard enough to become fitter or as fit as you could be. So it is important that you know what your target zone is and keep checking – until you have a good idea of how much or how little you need to do – whether you are staying within it when you exercise.

To calculate the right rate for you, first subtract your age from 220. That, in theory, is your maximum heart rate, and it is unwise ever to push yourself beyond it. Now subtract your resting pulse from your maximum heart rate, to give your maximum pulse gap. When you are exercising at maximum efficiency, your pulse should be between 50 and 75 per cent of that gap plus your resting pulse rate. Go higher, and you get diminishing returns.

Checking your pulse during and immediately after exercise not only ensures that you stay within the most efficient training zone for you, but also gives you instant feedback on how your fitness is improving. You will find, in time, that as you become fitter you have to work harder or longer before you get your pulse up into the zone in which you want it to stay for between 20 and 30 minutes in order to improve your stamina further. How quickly your pulse drops again at the end of strenuous exercise is another measure of how fit you are, and you might also like to check your resting pulse rate from time to time. That may also go down as you become fitter.

Before you start

When you have chosen your exercise programme – the next chapter will give you further help to do that – and you are ready to go, there are a few more pitfalls it would pay to watch out for:

- Don't try to do too much too soon. It is tempting, once you have made the resolution, to go all-out for results, but if you push yourself too hard, you may burn out and give up – or worse, you may injure yourself and have to stop exercising completely for weeks or even months while you heal. In addition, your body does need days off to rest up and recover.

- Don't underdo it either. Anything you do to become more active – using stairs instead of lifts, for example – helps. But the ideal towards which you need to work if you *really* want results is at least three to five aerobic workouts lasting 20 to 30 minutes a week.

- Keep the intensity moderate. It does not help improve your fitness if your heart rate is not high enough, or if it is too high.

- Never skip your warm-up or cool-down and your starting and finishing stretches (see under Get stretched, below). Warming up by starting slowly and carefully, and stretching your muscles gently before you start exercising vigorously, will lessen the risk of injury. Cooling down by exercising more slowly for the last five minutes of the session ensures that the changes in your cardiovascular system during strenuous exercise are not reversed too abruptly – important for everyone and particularly if you know you have a heart problem. (If you do have a heart problem, be sure to talk to your doctor about any exercise before you start.) Those final stretches also help rid the muscles of the waste material that builds up in them during strenuous exercise which can make you feel stiff and sore later.

- If you suffer back pain, the warm-up is doubly important, as is the kind of exercise you choose to do. Everyone exercising – but especially those with back problems – should avoid bending forward, touching the toes, raising both legs at the same time while lying on the floor, twisting the body or working with legs straight and knees locked. (For more about exercising with a bad back, see the Which? Consumer Guide *Understanding Back Trouble*★★.)

- Make sure your clothes are comfortable. You don't need designer gear. You probably don't even need to buy anything new, but whatever you wear should be unrestricting and comfortable. Natural fibres that breathe are particularly good.

- Never mask pain by taking pain-killers in order to carry on exercising. That's a shortcut to serious injury.

- Don't get straight into a hot bath or sauna after strenuous exercise if you have circulation problems such as varicose veins or raised blood pressure. It can make them worse.

- Remember if muscles feel a bit sore they are complaining about how you have neglected them in the past. But if they feel really painful, they are asking for mercy in the present. Stop if you feel pain, but if you are working aerobically, not too suddenly.

Get stretched

There is just one more vital consideration before you can embark on an exercise programme. It is important to protect your muscles by stretching them before you start any vigorous activity and again when you finish. If you have coaching in a sport, you may learn stretches particularly appropriate for it, and good classes include their own stretching routines.

Below are some general-purpose stretching exercises. They are a good all-round set to prepare you for aerobic exercise and can also be used to lengthen your muscles and rid them of waste products after it.

Do the first half conscientiously every time – ideally after a few minutes of comparatively gentle start-up activity to get your body warm – and you will minimise the risk of injury. Finish with the second half, following them with a few minutes more of gentle activity to allow your body to cool down at the end of your exercise session, and you are less likely to feel stiff later.

They are also a useful way to maintain suppleness. Everyone would benefit from working through the pre-exercise routine at least three times a week, even if not using them to prepare for aerobic exercise.

Warning: *Do all these standing poses with knees slightly bent to protect the back, never with legs so straight the knees are locked. Stretch only as far as is comfortable for you.*

Before

Arm circling: Stand tall and relaxed (and remember to keep knees slightly bent). Put your fingertips on your shoulders and circle your bent arms forwards 10 times. Reverse the direction and circle back for another 10.

Shoulder shrugs Still with bent knees, shrug your shoulders up towards your ears and down again 10 times. Then lift shoulders up and circle them to the back, down and to the front and up

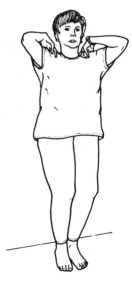

Arm Circling

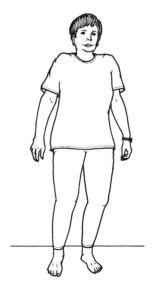

Shoulder Shrugs

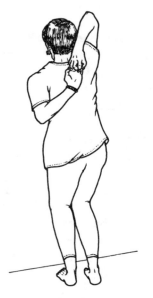

Arm Stretching

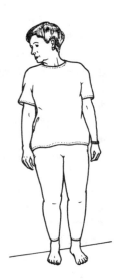

Neck Releasing

again half a dozen times; reverse direction for another six. You can do both sides together or one at a time, as you prefer.

Arm stretching: Take your left hand around the back of your waist, and move it up towards the base of you neck as far as you can comfortably, without straining. Take your right hand straight up in the air and stretch it up well, turn it so the palm faces the wall behind you, and then bend it and take it down your back to clasp the left hand if you can.

If you cannot reach, don't worry: you can hold an old belt in the hand that goes down your back and grasp it with the other across the gap. Work the hands along the belt towards one another as far as they will go without straining.

Reverse and repeat on the other side.

Neck releasing: Turn your head round to the right slowly and carefully as far as you comfortably can (don't strain). Bring it back to the centre and do the same on the other side. Repeat several times.

Then turn your head to the right, rotate it to bring your chin down on to your chest as far as you comfortably can, and then take it up again to the left. Repeat from left to right. Repeat both directions several times. (*Never* continue that rotation round the back. It crunches the spine.)

Torso twists: Put your fingertips together about collarbone height and take your elbows out to the sides so your arms are shoulder high and parallel with the ground. With feet hip-width apart and knees bent, turn your top half as far to the right as you can, while keeping your hips facing forward. Do the same on the other side. Repeat half a dozen times each side.

(If you find it difficult to keep your hips forward, try doing it sitting on a chair with your feet on the floor so your hips cannot move round – see illustration.)

Sideways bend: Stand with your feet a bit more than hip-width apart, your right leg turned out to the side, and your right knee bent. Take your left arm up over your head and put your right hand on your right leg, above the knee. Bend sideways over your right leg. Don't bend forwards or backwards; imagine you're between two walls. Don't strain or jerk. Go down gently, relax, and let gravity and your weight ease you further down. Keep your hips facing forward. If you can't, you are going down too far. Hold

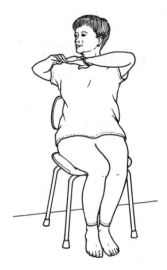

Torso Twists

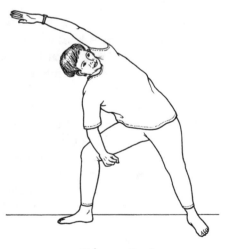

Sideways Bend

the stretch. Then come up carefully and repeat on the other side. Do a second stretch on each side.

Hamstring stretch 1: Standing up, bend the left knee and take the right leg forward. Turn the foot up so only the heel is on the ground. Bend forward and put both hands on the bent leg just a bit above (never on) the knee. If you don't immediately feel a good stretch right up the back of the straight leg, shift your weight forward further until you do. Do the other side.

Quad stretch: To stretch the quadriceps muscle, which runs right down the front of the top half of the leg, stand on one leg (with slightly bent knee), hold on to something for balance if you need to and bend the other leg up behind you. If you cannot feel a stretch down the front of the bent leg, keep your hips square on to the front and take the leg back a bit further until you can.

Calf stretch: Stand facing a wall with your hands on it and hips facing it square on. Bend one leg slightly and take the other leg back behind you. Ease the heel of the back leg down to the ground and press back into it. If you don't feel a good stretch in the calf, move the back leg further away from the wall and ease the heel down again until you do.

Repeat on the other side.

After
Hamstring stretch 2: This is a good one to do after you finish exercising (see illustration on p.34).

Lie on your back with your knees bent and feet on the floor. Take one bent leg and bring the knee towards the chest. Hold it with both hands (not at the knee), then gently ease it towards you as far as you comfortably can. (If your foot shakes, you are over-doing it – be sure to ease off.) Hold it there and relax it so only your hands are holding it (ideally it should be so relaxed that if you took your hands away the leg would flop to the floor). After a few seconds, you will probably find it will ease further towards your body. A few seconds later, try to ease it closer. When you have it as close to your body as it will go without straining or pulling, hold for 10 to 15 seconds. (Don't worry if it isn't very close.) Then do the other side.

Buttock stretch: Lie on your back on the floor again, this time with one foot on the floor. Cross the other leg over the bent one

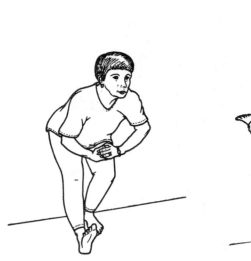

Hamstring Stretch 1

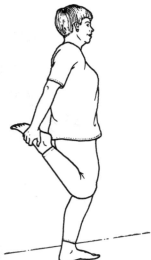

Quad Stretch

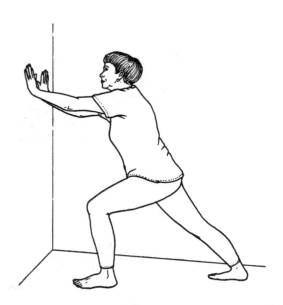

Calf Stretch

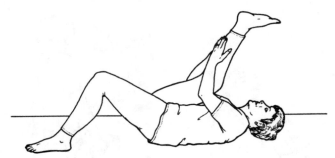

Hamstring Stretch 2

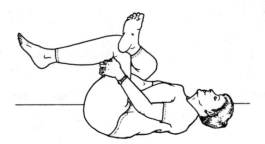

Buttock Stretch

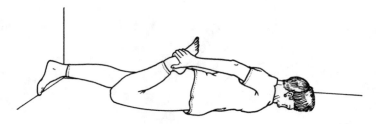

Quad Stretch

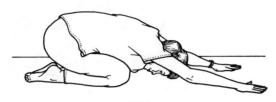

Yoga Child Pose

and lift the underneath leg towards you so it pulls the top leg up towards your body, too. Then do the other side. You can increase the stretch by using your hands to pull the bottom leg further towards you.

Quad stretch: While you are on the floor, do a quad stretch lying on your front and taking a leg at a time up behind you (as if you were doing the standing version, but rotated through 90 degrees). Make sure your head and hips remain on the floor.

Yoga child pose: Sit back on your heels, stretch your arms really well up above you, and bend forward so your arms and upper body are reaching out along the floor. Hold for 15 seconds.

Follow with **arm circling, shoulder shrugs, neck releasing** and **calf stretches** again as above.

All that remains now is for you to discover the right activity or activities for you. The next chapter will help you decide.

CHAPTER 2

WHICH EXERCISE?

IF YOU do want to take the plunge and set out to become fitter, how do you choose the best activity or exercise for you? Here are a number of tips to help you reduce your shortlist and ensure that you make the safest approach to your chosen activity:

- Find a type or, even better, types of exercise you really enjoy. If you approach exercising in the spirit of taking the medicine, you might start with a flurry of determination, but it will not be long before you give it up.
- The right exercise for you is not only something you enjoy doing but also something that really leaves you feeling good. That means it will be much easier to get going next time.
- If you are new to exercise, start gently and take your time building up.
- If you are not used to vigorous activity at all, you might want to check with your doctor before you start so that what you plan is appropriate, even if you believe you are in good health. This is particularly advisable if you are over 65.
- You should check with your doctor if you have had chest pains, high blood pressure or heart disease, asthma, bronchitis, back trouble, joint pains, diabetes, or if you are recovering from an illness or operation.
- If you overdo it at first, for example by going straight into playing squash without having built your fitness level up gradually, it could be very bad for your heart. What is more likely, however, is that if you don't start gently enough, you will injure joints or muscles, or just end up stiff and sore.
- Although you should start gently, if you really want to improve your stamina, you should aim to build up eventually to 20 or 30

minutes of exercising quite strenuously two or three times a week.

- Consider the cost. It is better to be realistic about what you can afford rather than jump in at the deep end and be disappointed to find you cannot keep it up.
- Financial restrictions are no excuse for not exercising at all. Walking and running are free, and many other sports, including swimming, can be quite inexpensive.
- Shop around. Some local authorities provide inexpensive facilities for many sports. Some public pools and private health clubs with gyms, pools, tennis courts and other facilities offer reduced rates for older members or reductions if you can go off-peak. Ask about season tickets, too.
- If you find it hard to make time for exercise, remind yourself how much more energy that exercise will give you. It might take an effort, but it is good time management as well as health management to build exercise into your life.
- Decide whether you want your exercise to be something sociable – done where you enjoy the company of other people – or something you will be quite happy to do on your own. Or you may choose a little of each.
- Exercise shouldn't cause muscle pain. If it does, stop.
- If you feel pain in the chest, neck or upper left arm, stop.
- If you find exertion seems to keep bringing on even vague chest pains, check with your doctor before you continue – sooner rather than later.
- You cannot hope to increase your stamina without becoming puffed and sweaty. Breathless is okay; speechless means you have gone too far.
- Stop if you feel dizzy or faint or break out in a cold sweat. If it keeps happening or you do faint during exercise, see your doctor.
- If you feel ill or have a cold or flu, it is better not to exercise until you feel well again.
- Don't exercise after any illness for which you have had to consult your doctor until he or she approves your starting again.
- Wait at least two hours after you eat a meal before exercising.
- Don't exercise after you have been drinking alcohol.

- Don't exercise in extremely hot or extremely cold conditions.
- Consider how you are going to cover all three essential components of fitness in your exercise programme – stamina, suppleness and strength. You might decide you want to combine different types of exercise, which also has the advantage of lessening the chance of overdoing any particular type of exertion. The chart on p.40 shows how different sports rate in terms of each of those fitness dimensions.

You might, for example, decide to start by walking briskly on the level, which has some effect on stamina but not much on suppleness and strength, and taking a class in yoga, to help keep you supple. Then, when walking has increased your fitness enough, you might want to add in a weekly game of tennis or badminton, both of which have some effect on all three elements of overall fitness. Or, if you are already quite fit and looking to improve, you might want to jog or walk uphill briskly, really pumping your arms as you go for stamina, and do yoga for suppleness and weight-training for strength. Or you might decide to swim regularly. Once you build up to swimming quite hard, you are following one of the few exercise regimes that rate highly on all three aspects of fitness (though, as you will see below, it is not all it might be for preserving bones).

Another option is to join a health club with a good gymnasium and well-trained staff who will assess your start-up status, work out a programme for you that will increase your all-round fitness at a safe rate, monitor your progress and upgrade the programme regularly to meet your changing needs.

You might decide to start walking or cycling to work if that is feasible in your circumstances, a choice which also gets economic and ecological brownie points. Of course, increased activity does not have to be an all-or-nothing affair. It can help, too, if you make minor life-style changes such as not always getting out of the car for journeys short enough to walk, and using the stairs rather than automatically getting in a lift.

Here, to help you decide what's right for you, are some further details of what is involved in different activities.

Table 1: ACTIVITY RATING

Activity	Stamina	Suppleness	Strength	Comment
Aerobics	★★★	★★★	★★	A lot depends on the teacher; can be pricey
Badminton	★★	★★	★★	Most sports centres have courts
Circuit training	★★★	★★★	★★★	A lot depends on the quality of the routine/ class
Climbing stairs	★★	★	★★	You don't need a gym
Cricket	★	★★	★	Sociable; find a club
Cycling (hard)	★★★	★	★★	Wear a helmet
Dancing (ballroom)	★	★★	★	Good for co-ordination
Dancing (disco)	★★	★★	★	Not just for the young
Digging the garden	★	★	★★★	Mind your back
Golf	★	★★	★	Start by taking lessons
Jogging	★★★	★	★	Use grass, not road; wear proper shoes
Rope-skipping	★★★	★★	★	Not just for boxers
Rounders	★★	★	★★	Or try soft-ball
Rowing	★★★	★	★★	Mind your back
Soccer	★★	★★	★★	Keep on running
Squash	★★★	★★★	★★	Wait till you're fit
Swimming (hard)	★★★	★★★	★★★	Best all-round
Tennis	★★	★★	★★	Find all-weather courts
Walking/rambling	★★	★	★	Hill walks can score ★★ for strength
Weight training	★	★★	★★★	Make sure you're properly supervised
Yoga	★	★★★	★	Start in a class

KEY: ★★★ Very good. ★★ Some effect. ★ Little or no effect.
Your skill and how hard you play will also affect the rating.

The options

Aerobics can build stamina and help maintain bone mass, vital for women around the menopause and beyond. Exercising with others to music can also be great fun. To avoid injury, it is crucial to find a good teacher. Check that he or she is qualified. Be wary if a teacher never or rarely corrects anyone's technique in class, or if s/he lets people join the class late without warming up. Expect a gentler cool-down section at the end of the class and for the strenuous middle segment to be sandwiched between before-and-after stretching. Classes often include some floor work for muscle strength towards the end. Most places will let you watch a class before joining up.

Expect a good teacher to ask or recognise who is new to the class and check whether new people have any injuries or health problems. It is a plus if the teacher expects you to take your pulse two or three times during the class. Look also for someone who encourages questions and is always happy (and able) to explain why they do what they do.

Find out what level of fitness the class is aimed at. Is it suitable for beginners? Is it high or low impact, or a mixture of both? High impact means lots of running on the spot and/or jumping up and down, which can endanger joints, especially if done on a hard floor. Low impact keeps a foot on the floor, which means less impact on joints. Some teachers give high- and low-impact options all the way through the class. Low impact does not necessarily mean low intensity, though. You will find you can work up quite a glow with high-intensity, low-impact aerobics.

If you are getting uncomfortably out of breath, don't try to keep up with the rest of the class. Slow down, but keep moving gently. (A good teacher should see that you don't stop moving completely.) How safe an aerobics class is depends not only on how good the teacher is and how up-to-date his or her training, but also on the type of floor (especially for high-impact work). The best is sprung; the worst is concrete. Some classes are too large for a teacher to be able to watch individuals carefully, although good mirrors – and experience – help.

Aqua-aerobics has all the advantages of the cardiovascular, leg and upper body workout you get from aerobics, but because body weight is supported by water, there is not the same potentially damaging impact on joints. This makes it a particularly useful option for people who are overweight or have orthopaedic or back problems. Working against the resistance of the water can enhance the muscle-strengthening effect, too.

Because your weight is supported by water and not subjected to the force of gravity, aqua-aerobics is not efficient at building and retaining the structural strength in bones. But being supported by the water makes it safer for anyone whose bones are already weakened through osteoporosis. Not all pools have classes, however, and classes tend to be extremely popular where they are available, making them crowded or difficult to join.

Badminton is one of the most popular sports in the UK. It is a sociable game, can be played at all levels and by all age groups, and is excellent for building power and stamina. Badminton strengthens the muscles in the back, shoulders, arms and legs, and the better you become at it the more energetic the game becomes and so the greater the benefit.

If you have a back problem, however, it could be a bit risky to play badminton, since the sport requires bending and twisting. Badminton is not expensive. All the equipment you need is shoes, racket and shuttlecock. There are centres, clubs and halls all over the country where it is played. Most don't have a dress code; anything comfortable goes. You can hire a racket to try before you buy. To get started, find out about local venues (your public library should know), and also whether there are local classes where you can improve your technique.

Bowls is not a big stamina builder, but it can help improve flexibility in your arms and shoulders, make your legs stronger and enhance hand-eye co-ordination and concentration. It can be played indoors or out. You need flat, smooth-soled shoes (to protect the greens), and clubs can be strict about dress. You can hire woods (bowls) to see if you like it before you splash out on your own. Bowls can put a strain on a bad back.

Circuit training, like aerobics, depends for its effectiveness largely on the ability of the teacher and the routine he or she devises. It is stamina training, and consists of a series, or 'circuit', of exercises done in sequence. Some of the exercises may involve using gym equipment. If you find a good class, circuit training is one of the rare activities that can rival swimming by scoring a 'very good' on stamina, suppleness and strength. Read the tips under the section on Aerobics, above, to help you find a good teacher.

Cycling can be done outdoors, provided you have somewhere safe to ride, preferably away from heavy traffic; or it can be done indoors on a stationary bike. It is best if you are starting cycling outdoors to do it on Sundays, when the roads are quieter, or to look for cycle lanes in parks. As cycling keeps the weight off load-bearing joints, cyclists are less prone to ankle and knee injuries than joggers or runners. If you cycle hard for long enough, your stamina will increase and you will burn up calories. Good warm-up exercises for it will help keep you supple, too. Some stationary bikes have a dual action that works both the upper and lower body at the same time.

To cycle outside, start on the flat and keep a comfortable pace for about five miles and see how you cope with that. Increase gradually when you are ready. Protect yourself from serious head injuries by wearing a helmet that carries a British Standard Kite-mark. When *Which?* magazine tested 11 cycling helmets that didn't carry the British Kitemark (results published in the August 1991 issue), it found that only three of them reached an acceptable standard.

Important points to bear in mind when buying a helmet include:

- Buy the smallest size of helmet that is a comfortable, snug fit on you. When you have it on without the buckle done up, it should touch the head at the crown, sides, back and front at the same time. If it doesn't, try a size down.
- Most helmets come with sizing pads that you can then use to make the final adjustments to fit.
- Don't buy a helmet that restricts your vision or hearing.
- If you have an accident, buy a new helmet, even if the old one does not look at all damaged.

You might want an anti-pollution mask, too, unless you are lucky enough to make your journeys where the air is relatively clean. When you are exercising and breathing heavily in a polluted atmosphere, chemicals can get deeper into your lungs. Although smoke and sulphur dioxide levels have dropped dramatically since the 1956 Clean Air Act, we are only beginning to look at the problem of other air pollutants. Breathing in mixtures of them may cause problems which we don't know much about yet.

You can hire a bike for a few rides before you splash out on one of your own, if you want to be sure that cycling is for you. Machines do tend to be expensive to buy, although you might find what you want secondhand, and once you have a bike it is cheap to maintain. If you are buying, choose a saddle for your usual riding position. Thin racing saddles let your legs move freely when leaning forward. Conventional, fatter saddles suit the more upright position on some mountain bikes and small-wheeled bikes. Some manufacturers make wider 'ladies' saddles. Some shops will change the saddle if you don't like the one fitted to the bike you are buying.

For more comprehensive advice on everything from choosing a bike to maintaining, insuring and securing it safely whenever you leave it, see the August 1991 issue of *Which?* magazine. If you find you are really keen and want to tour or race, there are plenty of groups and clubs you could join. Some also arrange outings, weekends away and cycling holidays. If you use your bike as transport as well as for exercise, cycling can be self-financing, even money-saving.

When *Which? way to Health* magazine (February 1992) tested home exercise bikes, it found that only three models out of eleven put through tough laboratory tests by the Association of Consumer Research survived them unscathed (although some developed more serious problems than others). Of the three most highly rated models, the least expensive cost £160, nearly £100 more than the cheapest in the test, and another was the most expensive bike in the test, priced at £245.

An equally disappointing finding was that, although almost two-thirds of people surveyed used their home exercise bikes regularly when they first had them, just over half had stopped using them or used them less than once a month after a time. Only just over one-quarter of long-term owners still used the bikes three times a week or more.

So before you decide to buy a home exercise bike, you need to be sure you will continue to use it. It might help if you can set it up so that you can watch television while you pedal, or get into the habit of bicycling to your favourite radio programme. If you do decide to buy, the points to consider are:

- **Resistance:** The bike must give you something to pedal against. You need to be able to set a low level for warming up and cooling down, and a higher, constant level for a steady workout; and to increase the higher level over time as you become fitter.
- **Endurance:** Not yours this time, the machine's. You want it to last a reasonable length of time and stand up to the wear and tear of regular use.
- **Safety:** You want to be sure it is not going to fall over or collapse while you are on it.

Whether you are cycling indoors or out, don't forget to stretch before you start and after you finish. Be sure to sandwich a strenuous effort against high resistance between four or five minutes of more gentle cycling at either end of the exercise period, in order to warm up your muscles before you get going and to cool them down again afterwards.

Dancing can be a good way to keep fit, with the bonus of being a sociable activity, too. It is difficult to be too specific about the exact contribution dancing will make to each of the different elements of fitness because it comes in so many varieties. Generally, however, the more energetically you throw yourself into it, the more it will built stamina and protect bones. It will also build strong legs, keep you supple and aid balance, co-ordination and concentration.

You will find classes suitable for beginners in many types of dance to give you the chance to try it out. If you find ballroom isn't your forte, don't give up. That still leaves tap, ballet, contemporary, Latin American, jazz, jazz ballet, Scottish, Irish, clog, morris, sequence, disco and so on.

Costs vary. Private tuition may be on the pricey side, but there are local-authority classes, too. What you will need in the way of special clothes and shoes will also vary from class to class. Find out before you sign up. There are also classes in dance exercise – working out to music with longer and more complex routines than in an ordinary keep-fit or aerobics class.

Exercise bikes are discussed above under Cycling.

Exercise classes can be anything from gentle stretching to keep you supple to really tough cardiovascular aerobic workouts. Two considerations apply right across the range. First, make sure you know just what level and what type of exercise you are letting yourself in for before you make a commitment. Second, make sure you find a good teacher. (See tips about selecting one under Aerobics, above.)

One series of classes set up under the Department of Health's 'Look After Your Heart/Look After Yourself' programme solves the 'appropriate levels' problem by organising the classes so that different people work at different levels under expert supervision at the same time. The classes cover not only exercise but also healthy eating and other life-style issues, as well as the issue of recognising and dealing with stress. To find the one nearest you, contact the HEA Business Unit*.

Fitness walking is discussed under Power walking, below.

Golf is a sport that appeals right across the age range. More young people are taking it up than ever before, and at the other end of the scale there are people who still play well into their 80s and credit golf with keeping them not only physically but also mentally on the ball.

You can try it out without spending too much. Many local authorities now have golf courses, although you may find they charge £10 or more a round. You can hire clubs until you know if golf is really going to be for you. Some parks also have putting greens or 'pitch 'n putts', where you can try out some aspects of the game, and there are driving ranges where you can pay for a bucket of balls to practise with. Private clubs, most local-authority courses and some driving ranges have professionals from whom you can book lessons. It is usually cheaper to book for a number of sessions.

Courses vary considerably in how strenuous they are to play, and the speed at which a golfer moves between shots is also important in determining how much the game contributes to stamina. Even the combination of speediest and toughest, however, will do more for suppleness than for stamina or strength.

Golf does strengthen the back and shoulders, and maintains spine rotation, which is necessary for a fit back. But people with back problems may find that sudden, jerky movements when swinging a club can make things worse. The secret of golf can be found not in brute strength but in co-ordination, timing and concentration. It can be relaxing – although a round on a bad day can leave a golfer feeling more stressed and/or depressed than when he or she teed off. And golfing in Japan, where just getting far enough up the corporation ladder to enable you to get on to a golf course at all can be a lifetime's ambition, proves that the relationship between the game and stress is not as simple as it is sometimes painted – as you will discover at the end of Chapter 7.

The main drawback is that if you get hooked and decide you want to buy the equipment and join a private club, you will undoubtedly find that golf is either expensive or very expensive, depending partly on where you live. It can be difficult to get into a club where you don't know members, and clubs in some parts of the country may have long waiting lists and may restrict admission to people who already hit a pretty respectable ball.

Jogging is the slowest pace at which you can run. It costs nothing but the price of a good pair of shoes, and is convenient because you can do it whenever and wherever it suits you. Jogging jars less if it's done on grass than on roads or hard pavements, although grass is often less even, making ankle-twisting more of a risk. So if you do jog on grass, look where you are going. If you must run on roads at night, wear light-coloured clothes and reflective bands.

If you can walk three miles in 45 minutes, you are ready to jog. If you haven't had much exercise recently or you are new to jogging, start by mixing walking and jogging for short, fixed distances. That's a better strategy than jogging until you are so fatigued you must slow down to a walk. Gradually increase the proportion of jog-to-run until you can jog for the whole distance, for up to 20 minutes. Don't go over 20 minutes in total before you can jog the whole of that time. Once you can, you can gradually increase the time to 30 minutes.

Here are some tips on how you should jog:

- Have your arms bent at the elbow, with wrists and fingers relaxed and loose, forearm roughly parallel to the ground and hands brushing past your abdomen as you run.

- Jog tall and upright and avoid leaning forward. Keep your head up and your back straight and look ahead of you, not down at your feet.
- Keep your stride short and easy.
- Breathe deeply and rhythmically.
- Don't run on your toes or you will strain your calf muscles. Try to learn to land with the weight mostly on the heel and then roll the weight forward through the foot so you are on the ball before you take off again, pushing off with your toes.
- If you find you are getting soreness, try to give more at the knees, so you can learn to land with your whole foot on the ground, rather than coming down too much on your toes.

When you are fit enough, you can, if you want, speed up and move from jogging to running. (See Running, below.) Jogging can cause 'overuse' injuries to feet, knees, ankles and hips. If you start gently and keep off hard surfaces for lengthy periods, you shouldn't have serious problems. But if you have arthritis in legs, hips or back, or are overweight, you might be better off opting for a form of exercise such as cycling or swimming instead.

One of the advantages of jogging is that you can do it whenever and wherever it suits you, and it can also be sociable. Many clubs welcome new members and cater for all levels of abilities − or you can just arrange to jog with a friend.

Health clubs and gyms, if well run by properly trained staff, will devise a programme specifically for you and will monitor your fitness at regular intervals, so you know just how much progress you are making and when your programme needs to be changed. Attentive staff will also be quick to spot any exercise you are doing incorrectly and will tell you so, rather than risk letting you injure yourself.

Clubs often offer a wide variety of exercises under the same roof. Many combine resistance and weight-training machines and aerobic equipment in the gym, have assorted exercise classes (for which members are often given discounted rates), and also have a swimming pool and squash and tennis courts. Members thus can have a varied exercise programme under one roof and can ring the changes to keep boredom at bay. (See also Weight training, below.)

To select a club:

- Ask to have a good look-round beforehand.
- Make sure you go at the time of day you would want to use it, so you can see how crowded it is. (Be wary if you are told inspections are only arranged at certain times.)
- Have a look at the state of the equipment. How new is it? Does it look well-maintained? Is there plenty of space between pieces of apparatus?
- Ask plenty of questions to ascertain whether the staff seem knowledgeable and helpful.
- Is there a lively and interested atmosphere? Notice boards can be revealing. Are they bright and informative? Or home to a few tired old announcements and yellowing cuttings?
- Ask other members about the club.

Health clubs are often expensive, but before you let that deter you if you want to join one, ask about off-peak and/or age-related deals.

Hiking, also known as walking or rambling, can mean anything from a short gentle stroll on the flat to long, fast, strenuous hill walking that needs – and builds – plenty of leg strength and stamina. How good it is for you depends on how long and how hard you do it. Hikers might start with a mile or two and build up to walking steadily all day, but even walking the dog more briskly or walking to the shops rather than driving is a start.

The equipment you need also depends on how long you are going to be out, and in what conditions and at what time of the year. Always carry a sweater if you are going high, even in the middle of summer. In winter, think in terms of clothes that keep out the damp and wind as well as the cold, or you could be caught out by the wind-chill factor. If you are out for hours in winter and you aren't properly dressed for it, hypothermia is a real danger. Layers of thin clothes are warmer than one layer of thick. A warm hat to prevent heat loss from your head and gloves or mitts are essential.

Carry extra clothes, food and drink in a backpack. Put in a torch, especially in winter, if there is even the remotest chance you will still be out after dark. You can buy very lightweight survival blankets, too, that will fold so small they can go in a pocket. They can be invaluable to keep an injured person warm until help arrives or to treat hypothermia. Take a first-aid kit for bites, cuts, blisters and sprains. It is sensible always to let someone know where you are going and when you are due back – essential if you are going alone.

You can walk over dry, gentle countryside in summer in any sturdy shoe, but for rougher terrain or winter walking you need proper walking boots with a deep tread. Good specialist shops will help you choose the ones most suitable for you and the use for which you intend them. Many will allow you to wear them around at home for several days and return them (as long as they are unmarked and you have the receipt) if they are not proving comfortable. (Check that before you buy.)

Nowadays, boots can be tough and have a thick tread and still be remarkably light. Wear them over two pairs of socks to minimise blisters. You want a thin pair next to the skin, and a thicker pair outside that. Cotton is ideal for the inner ones and wool for the outer. Always break in new shoes or boots before a long walk.

The countryside is criss-crossed with footpaths and bridleways where you are free to walk. They are usually well signposted, and there are plenty of maps and guidebooks on the market. These include books of circular walks which tell you where you can park your car to start, and give you a route that will bring you back to it. A compass in your pocket could well prove helpful.

If you want to walk in company, or to have the chance to learn the lore from more experienced walkers, contact the countrywide Ramblers' Association* or any local walking group. A number of organisations do holidays in which hikers set out each day carrying only lunch in a backpack, while the organisers move their luggage from place to place for them. If you want your walking hard and fast for more concentrated stamina-building, see Power walking, below.

Home fitness equipment includes (besides exercise bikes, discussed under Cycling, above) treadmills, rowing machines, stair-climbing machines and various strength-training items. In fact, most of what is available in a well-equipped gym can be installed in your home. It is convenient to have it there because cutting out travelling enables you to get full value out of the time you have available for exercise. It is always wise to try before you buy.

Good exercise equipment is expensive, and not everyone has enough room to house it. Having only one item saves space but limits you to a less varied and healthy programme and can be boring. Using the equipment at home also means there is no one on hand to train you in correct use as in a well-run gym, or to keep an eye on you in case mistakes creep into your technique.

A good rowing machine works upper- and lower-body muscles, and provides an excellent cardiovascular workout with a minimum of stress on hip and knee joints and no impact on other joints. But it may be less kind to the lower back, and a good one will be expensive.

Treadmills enable you to walk, jog or run indoors on a moving belt and provide all the benefits of doing the same exercise outside, except that there is slightly less impact stress. However, they take up a lot of room and a really good, reliable one is extremely expensive.

Stair-climbers work leg and buttock muscles and give you a moderate cardiovascular workout, but can be hard on knees, hips, lower back and ankles. They vary widely in price and quality. The more you spend, the better you get. If your balance is good and you have stairs at home, you could always climb them instead.

Home equipment does not always have to cost a fortune, however. One economy item that can make a major contribution to stamina is a skipping rope.

Keep-fit classes are another sociable way to get fit. Like aerobics (see above), how good a class is depends largely on the quality of the teaching. Classes should give all your muscles a workout to increase strength and include plenty of joint moving for flexibility. The amount of stamina-building varies from class to class. Find out what the class aims to do and what fitness level it caters for before you start. Some local authorities include keep-fit in their adult education programmes and/or have health centres where classes might be less expensive than private ones, although there are often very inexpensive classes in clubs, church halls and community centres.

Orienteering is rallying on legs. Participants jog through forests and woods and on common land, following a route by reading a map and using a compass as they go. The sport is highly organised, with everything from simple courses for beginners to international meetings. It is suitable for a wide range of ages, and whole families go in for it.

If it appeals to you, the best way to get started is by contacting an orienteering club. You don't need a lot of speed, though if you are an out-and-out beginner or have recently returned to exercise, you might want to build up your jogging a bit on your own first.

Personal trainers are becoming increasingly popular. On the plus side, because they don't have a whole class on which to concentrate, they can tailor a programme that is exactly right for you. Personal trainers can be excellent for motivation, and will reassess and redesign your programme regularly. (And you cannot slack off at the back of a class.)

On the minus side, you may have to search to find the right trainer. Look at Aerobics, above, for hints on selecting a teacher, and you will find most of them also apply here. Ask around your area for recommendations. If you know of someone who teaches classes as well as working one-to-one, you might join a class to see that person in action first. If you are going to be working on your own with a teacher in your home rather than in a class, it is even more important that you actually like and feel comfortable with him or her.

Another minus is the cost, although you may find some trainers who are willing to work with two or even more people in the same home for the same price or a small surcharge. So if you have the space and some like-minded local friends, you could share the expense.

Power walking means walking fast enough to get up a sweat; it is an ideal exercise for beginners and returners to exercise. Try level ground and avoid hills or walking into a strong wind when you start.

Walking aerobically offers all the benefits of jogging, cycling and aerobics, but without the risk of impact injury. It is weight-bearing exercise, important for building and maintaining bone mass, but kinder to bones that have already begun to thin than is jogging or running. In addition, the more you get your arms pumping, the more of a cardiovascular workout walking becomes.

Walking hard – so you can still carry on a limited conversation but are moderately out of breath – is enough aerobic exercise for many. Aim to be able to walk without stopping for about three miles in 45 to 55 minutes. You will still need to add in something for flexibility to make an ideal all-round programme. Don't forget to stretch before you start.

You may think you may already know how to walk. But here are a few points on technique to help you do it better:

- Keep your shoulders back, but relaxed.
- Chest out.
- Eyes ahead.
- Chin up.
- Swing your arms in rhythm with your step.
- Come down more on the heel of your foot and gradually roll the weight forward along the outer edge of the sole to the ball of the foot.
- Push off again with the toes.

For those looking for more demanding exercise – while still avoiding the injury risks to joints and muscles entailed by jogging – step up your walking by going faster, uphill, and pumping the arms more vigorously as you go.

Although walking carrying weights increases the energy burned up and can boost muscle strength, weights do interfere with the body's natural balance and rhythm – and that can make walking less enjoyable. Carrying hand weights while walking can also raise blood pressure, so could be dangerous for some people. Increasing speed and arm action to enhance the cardiovascular effects of walking, plus following the walk with some high-repetition, low-weight training for muscle strength, may be a better strategy.

Walking is free. All you need to get started is a pair of good shoes (see p.59). You can do it just about anywhere, anytime.

Rambling is discussed under Hiking, above.

Running is not for beginners. Start with walking if you are out of condition, and jog before you run. Running is a good cardiovascular workout that increases stamina and strength in the muscles in the calves, thighs and abdomen, but does little for flexibility. There is also a risk of damage to feet and legs.

If you want to improve leg power and stamina, don't always run the same speed and distance, but vary your routine with sprints, hill running, bursts of speed and interval training (which combines jogging with bursts of running hard).

Here are some tips on running technique:

- Relax your upper body. Your shoulders should not twist or rotate as you stride. Relax your arms and check from time to time if you need to unclench your fists.
- If the horizon seems to be moving up and down, it means you are bouncing and you need to shorten your stride a little. Too long a stride means your foot actually checks your momentum each time it lands.
- Your foot should come down fairly flat and directly under your hips.
- Keep your head up and eyes ahead. You breathe better and feel better if you do.
- Buy good shoes at a specialist shop where the staff know about running. They can check (by perhaps asking you to do a 'test walk' in talcum powder sprinkled on paper, or by looking at shoes you've already 'worn in') for any peculiarities in your technique (such as rolling your feet either in or out), and suggest shoes to minimise the effect.

Squash is too strenuous a game to use to start with when you are trying to get fit. Play it only if you already really are. Most doctors discourage anyone over 50 taking up squash for the first time. For those fit enough for it, however, squash is excellent for stamina and suppleness, and has some effect on strength.

You can hire a racket to find out how much you like the game rather than buy one, although equipment is not particularly expensive, nor is playing at a local-authority leisure centre. But if you want to play at a private club, it could be costly.

Step aerobics is exercise done using a platform of variable heights to step on and off in a series of increasingly complicated manoeuvres as the class becomes more advanced. It is low-impact (explained under Aerobics, above) but can be quite high-intensity, even at beginner level, and increasingly so as step height and speed are increased.

Even beginners usually add in some upper-body work, once they have got the hang of the basic routines. As a class becomes more advanced, the routines become more complicated and the step platform higher. The upper-body work increases the stamina-building potential of step aerobics as well as its value as an all-round upper- and lower-body muscle workout. It particularly strengthens muscles in thighs, calves and buttocks, and improves co-ordination.

One of its advantages is that it is not difficult to learn in a beginners' class, while the increasing concentration it requires to move up through the levels makes it more mentally interesting than other comparable forms of exercise. Another advantage is that it can be better than high-impact aerobic workouts for people with bladder problems.

As with other aerobics classes, the most important safety factor is finding a good teacher who knows the correct technique and is quick to spot and inform anyone not following it. (See under Aerobics, above.) It is particularly important that the whole foot goes on the step every time. Heels should not be left hanging off the platform. Be concerned if a teacher does not explain that to beginners and fails to keep reminding and watching throughout the class.

Step aerobics tends to be a little more expensive than other aerobics classes since the correct equipment is not cheap. Because this kind of exercise is popular, classes often tend to be fully booked well in advance. You can buy your own step and work to a home video, but the British School of Osteopathy has reported injuries from step aerobics, sometimes from people overdoing it at classes, but mostly from people doing step at home alone and omitting the vital warming-up and stretching exercises. *Step Ahead with Carolan Brown* was given good safety ratings by the *Which? way to Health* survey discussed under Videos, below.

Stretching is not only essential to prepare muscles for strenuous exercise and to expel waste from them and lengthen them again after exercise, but also has benefits, particularly in improving flexibility, in its own right. You will find stretch classes in leisure centres, health clubs and local-authority programmes. The tips for finding a good teacher under Aerobics, above, can be helpful again here. Stretching also plays a major role in yoga. If you want to go it alone, the subject is dealt with exhaustively in *Soft Exercise, Complete Book of Stretching*★★ by Arthur Balaskas and John Stirk.

Swimming has the advantage that, because your weight is supported by water, there is no strain or impact on joints. This makes swimming particularly good for people with joint problems such as arthritis who need to keep their joints mobile without putting too much stress on them. It can also be helpful for people with asthma or bronchitis, and is a good starting point if you are considerably overweight.

Swimming gets a plus for being one of the few sports that is equally good for increasing stamina, suppleness and strength. However, because your weight is supported by water and so not subjected to the force of gravity, swimming is less efficient at building and retaining the structural strength in bones. For the same reason, however, it is safer for anyone whose bones are already weakened because of osteoporosis.

Some people find it boring to swim energetically up and down a pool for long enough to make swimming a worthwhile exercise. But for others, swimming is the time they get away from ringing telephones and demanding jobs and families, and just enjoy being alone with their thoughts. Many pools offer women-only sessions.

If you are doing crawl, it is better to take alternate breaths on opposite sides if you can because it is kinder to your neck. Breathe in through the mouth, out through the nose. People with back problems might want to have a word with their doctors before swimming, and should certainly avoid swimming with their heads up out of the water all the time. This puts a strain on the lower back.

Particularly if you are swimming for aerobic fitness, which means three or four good, hard sessions a week, it will pay you to use different strokes rather than sticking with one. You might like to warm up with breast stroke, move to crawl, then do some backstroke and finish off with breast stroke when you are starting to feel tired.

It is never too late to start. Many pools have lessons for different age groups, special reduced price sessions for over-50s, and season tickets to help keep the price down. The only other essential is a swimsuit, although many regular swimmers like to wear goggles which do protect eyes from possible soreness and infection. Some people like, as well, to wear a latex swimcap to protect hair and save having to dry it after every swim.

Table tennis is good for mobility and reflexes. How strenuous it is depends on how you hard and fast you play. It is an extremely sociable game and inexpensive. It does not need much in the way of equipment – just a bat and a ball and some comfortable clothes will do.

Like badminton (see above), it is played in sports centres, clubs and church halls, and there are classes at some clubs and some local-authority adult-education venues.

Tennis keeps shoulders, arms and legs supple and strong, and helps posture, balance, concentration and co-ordination. All that bending and stretching and leaping and running improves stamina, too. It is suitable for all ages and levels of fitness because it can be played at your own pace, as long as you find someone at about the same level to play with. Doubles is less strenuous than singles.

You can play on hard courts outdoors all year round, as long as the weather is kind, and more centres now have indoor facilities. You'll need tennis shoes and a racket and tennis balls, but these needn't cost the earth. A good sports shop will help you choose a racket which has the correct weight and the right-size grip for you.

What you need to wear depends upon where you play. Some clubs insist you wear all-white. If you find you enjoy tennis and want to improve your game, you can arrange coaching from the local professional or find out about local-authority classes in your area. Private clubs are more expensive and can be difficult to get into, but if you find you are becoming keen, you might want to try.

Videos for exercising at home are available to meet different fitness objectives and for people starting at different fitness levels. For example, some aim only to tone muscles and so improve the shape of part or all of the body. Others claim to increase aerobic fitness and help you lose weight. It is not always clear from the description on the box what the aim is, or how fit or experienced you have to be to use the video safely and successfully. If a friend owns a copy of the video you are thinking of buying, it would be useful to have a look at it first.

Home videos can really come into their own when people attend or have attended classes with good teachers and already know the basic dos and don'ts, and have good exercise technique. Even if the instruction on a video is clear and sensible, it cannot tell you – as a good teacher would – when you aren't getting it right.

A well-used video works out very much less expensive than going to regular classes, and it can be played whenever you have the time and the inclination. It can also supplement classes at holiday periods, when they tend to close down, or if your schedule is so erratic that you cannot always fit in with a class time-table.

However, when *Which? way to Health* magazine in its December 1992 issue asked a panel of experts to survey exercise videos, it found that not all the videos were as safe as they could be. Nor did it always say on the box if the exercises portrayed were unsuitable for beginners when the experts considered they were. Some videos were just plain out of date, using exercises that had been found to be unsafe and condemned by the experts years ago.

If you buy a video:

- Look for information about the fitness level at which you should be in order to start using it.
- See if it says it includes different levels of exercises, so that you can work harder with it as you get fitter.
- See what qualifications the instructor has. (This doesn't necessarily mean avoiding celebrity videos. *Cher Fitness: A New Attitude*, for example, leaves the instruction to an expert and got a high rating all round from *Which? way to Health*. On the other hand, the magazine panned *Chippendales: Muscle Motion* as apparently put together by someone who 'must have been living in a box for the last 10 years', and gave it an overall 'worst' rating.)
- Watch the video through before you try to join in, so you get to know the exercises. Pay particular attention to the safety tips.
- Watch the instructor closely and copy her or him – never the other participants.
- Don't skip the warm-up or cool-down, however short of time you are.
- Slow down for a while and then catch up again if you need to, and stop if you feel any pain.
- Always dress comfortably and wear suitable shoes.

Walking is covered under Hiking and Power walking.

Weight training can help keep you supple and make a major contribution to muscle and bone strength. It can be done with free weights or machines. Frequent repetition with light weights builds up stamina without making your body look huge and muscle-bound.

You can buy weights quite cheaply to use at home. You will find them in mail-order catalogues and advertised secondhand. It is important to learn correct techniques or you risk injury, especially to knees, shoulders and back. It pays to join a club or find a class run by your local authority or at a local sports centre.

Yoga teaches control of movement and breathing, and is excellent for suppleness and good for strengthening muscles, especially in the stomach, hips, thighs and back. However, it contributes little to stamina and needs to be part of an integrated programme to achieve all-round fitness.

There are many do-it-yourself books on yoga, but no matter how conscientiously you try to follow them, they are no substitute for a good teacher, at least at the start. It is very difficult to do yoga correctly on your own, but not difficult in most parts of the country to find a class. Private classes can be quite reasonable, or quite expensive. Local-authority yoga classes usually make a more modest charge.

If you want details of other sports or to contact the governing body of any sport, you can phone the **Sports Council's Information Centre** on 071-388 1277, or your local Sports Council Regional Office★.

The shoe for you

Having the right sports shoes can save you injuries. When your foot hits the ground, shock waves are transmitted to bones, muscles and joints. If you are running, your foot hits the ground with an impact equivalent to three times what you weigh. If you run a mile, your foot will hit the ground between 800 and 2000 times. Sports shoes are designed to absorb the shock of impact, preventing muscle, tendon and joint problems, and stress fractures. Over the long term, they aim to reduce the likelihood of osteoarthritis (inflammation of joints) or severe back pain.

Impact is not the only risk. Twisting and turning at speed, when you can lose your balance, can damage your legs. The risk of twisting or spraining an ankle is greater if you have the wrong shoe. A stiff-soled running shoe is not suitable for squash, where you need a more flexible sole for fast changes of direction. Also, if shoes don't fit, are not comfortable or don't support your feet the right way, you are asking for trouble.

Good sports shoes are expensive. Part of the reason is that they are in demand as status symbols, especially by the young. But part of the cost also reflects the research that has gone into them and the technology used to design and make them. When *Which? way to Health* tested a selection of cross-trainers (reported in the April 1991 issue), it found that the cheapest shoe did have disadvantages, but that paying much more didn't necessarily mean you got outstanding performance. It was found that running shoes tended to be most expensive and shoes for racket sports cheaper.

The survey found that most of the cross-trainers were suitable, as the manufacturers claimed, for more than one type of sport. But using cross-trainers did involve compromise. Generally, they were not as good for any particular sport as a shoe designed exclusively for use in that sport. They were not recommended for running long distances because the shock absorption in the heel is generally lower than it is in the best running shoes, and cross-trainers are heavier.

All sports shoes are best bought in specialist shops where you can expect expert advice. Here are some further tips for choosing shoes for different activities:

- **Running and jogging** need a shock-absorbing heel, good support all round, especially at the ankle, and good rough tread for outdoor running. Avoid shoes with a sole that flares out all round the heel because they could allow your feet to roll sideways. Instead of making you more stable, they could make it more likely you will end up twisting your ankle.

- For **tennis, squash and badminton and other racket sports**, you want quick changes of direction and to be able to swivel on the balls of your feet. Thin, flexible soles that are relatively flat, and shock-absorbent material under the ball of your foot, are required. You need support at the front of the foot. The grip you want depends on the sport and the surface on which you play it. You need, for example, to 'skid' a bit more in tennis. Avoid shoes with the back of the sole built up as much as a running shoe, and, again, the sole shouldn't be flared out.

- **Aerobics and keep-fit** shoes need good cushioning at the ball of the foot and heel. A high top is optional, but the shoe must be flexible and cut low at the back. Exercise classes often combine jogging, jumping and twisting. High tops support ankles, but you need a dip at the back for the Achilles tendon, which is at the back of the foot above the heel.
- **Cross-training** can be done most economically by choosing one shoe that is recommended by the manufacturer as suitable for all the activities you are combining. Although cross-trainers are expensive, a pair will still cost less than buying a different pair of shoes for each sport. However, the shoes will mean compromise – as noted above, they will probably not be quite as good for any one activity as shoes designed solely for use in that activity.
- **Weight training** requires a strong upper and side straps, and wide soles. Because lifting weights puts extra pressure on legs and feet, extra-stable shoes which stop you losing your balance are needed.

Whatever sport you are choosing shoes for, here are some additional general tips:

- Always try them. Don't rely on the given size, even if you have had the same brand before.
- Always try them with the type of socks with which you intend to wear them.
- Tie them right up and do up any straps to see how firmly they fit. The laces should come almost to the base of your ankle joint to give good support.
- Check the back of the heel. If it is high, rigid or digs into your heel, it could damage your tendon.
- Check that the sole is slightly higher at the heel than at the toe. That is the shape your feet are used to.
- Feel inside for seams that could rub your feet.
- Walk around in the shop to test their comfort. Bend your knees (keep them over your toes) and check that the shoes don't then feel too tight. Put all your weight on each foot in turn to make

sure the front of your foot has room to spread out. Wiggle your toes to make sure the shoes are deep enough.

- Crouch to check that the shoes will bend when your feet do.
- Make sure the shoe cups your heel firmly, and that your heel doesn't slip out as you walk.
- Check that your feet don't hang over the edges of the soles. That could make you unstable.
- Check the tread. You need a rough, durable one for outdoors and a smoother one for indoors.
- If the shoes feel painful or uncomfortable, leave them in the shop. If in doubt, don't buy.

A last word

If you were to begin to exercise vigorously and diligently today and keep it up for a year, some authorities estimate that by the end of that time you would have put the clock back 10 years. For as long as you keep up the regular exercise, you keep that 10-year bonus. Even if you are not prepared to make the commitment to getting up a sweat three times a week, any activity is better than none.

If exercise can make an enormous contribution to becoming and staying fit and healthy over 40, exercise combined with a healthy diet and not smoking (and avoiding passive smoking), provides the very best protection against the risk of serious illness such as heart disease.

A study in California reported in *The Lancet* (21 July 1990) put patients with angina and narrowing of the arteries on a life-style-changing regime in which they exercised for three hours a week, learned a series of stress-management techniques and stayed on a strict low-fat vegetarian diet without caffeine and with an alcohol limit of two units a day. The study found that the arteries of the patients on the regime actually widened over the course of a year. In the control group that did not make the changes, the condition continued to progress during that period. The patients who made the biggest changes to their life style also made the biggest improvements to the state of their arteries.

Only the most determined or motivated might be prepared to stick to such a regime rigidly enough to make disease actually regress. But most of us could benefit from simple changes to our diet to make it more healthy.

The next chapter considers what constitutes a sensibly healthy diet for the majority of us, and sets out how easily we can make improvements in what we eat.

CHAPTER **3**

HEALTHY EATING

A HEALTHY diet means eating in a way that gives us energy and vitality, and supplies us with everything our body needs to keep in good running order. It means eating to keep our immune systems in top working condition and to give us protection against conditions such as heart disease and cancers in which diet may be a factor. In fact, as we leave 40 behind, healthy eating becomes increasingly linked to maintaining a healthy heart and keeping to a sensible weight.

Healthy eating is not fanatical or faddish. It is about small everyday changes that make big differences in the long term. It is not about being a killjoy in the kitchen. When eating can no longer be a source of pleasure, we have lost something along the way. And healthy eating does not have to be hard work. Tinned baked beans on wholemeal toast is a very healthy meal.

Healthy eating is about choice. There are many, many ways to make what we eat more healthy. The trick is to select the ones that fit our tastes, preferences, purses and life styles – and figures, too. There are good health reasons, discussed in more detail later, not to allow ourselves to become seriously overweight.

Don't be put off if the topic of healthy eating seems to inspire a glut of advice. The aim of this chapter is to offer a broad understanding of the underlying principles, followed by options from which to select the ones that are right for you. Healthy eating is about variety and pleasure – with the emphasis not on giving up, but rather on finding other ways.

Nor is it suggested that you change the way you eat overnight. If, when you have read this chapter, you do feel your diet is in need of a fairly extensive overhaul, it is better to make changes slowly, one or two at a time. That way, you will gradually establish a new and permanent healthy-eating pattern for you and your family – rather than revolution one week, relapse the next.

The guidelines

The World Health Organization (WHO) made diet recommendations based on research into nutrition and disease prevention in 1990. Its report, 'Diet, Nutrition, and the Prevention of Chronic Disease', was written by a panel of international scientists brought together specifically to review the whole body of nutritional research. They concluded that what we do and don't eat:

- can help prevent coronary heart disease, hypertension, stroke, gallstones, tooth decay and obesity
- can give some protection against cancer
- may contribute to osteoporosis, diabetes in middle age, and intestinal and bowel problems.

The Committee on Medical Aspects of Food Policy (COMA) made its own assessment of the current state of knowledge, particularly as it is relevant to the UK, and published its recommendations the following year.

The combined guidelines, which are for a healthy diet for healthy people, are quite straightforward and are set out below. (If you already have heart disease, your doctor may put you on a more restrictive regime, particularly in relation to fats. Other illnesses and diseases may also mean that you will require special dietary requirements.)

Fruit and vegetables
The WHO recommends that we eat at least five portions of fruit and vegetables (other than potatoes) a day. It doesn't matter whether the vegetables are frozen or the fruit canned, though if you choose cans it is better to avoid added salt or sugar, and opt for fruit in fruit juice rather than a sugar syrup.

Carbohydrates
COMA recommends we should get nearly half our daily calories from complex carbohydrates found in starchy foods such as

breads, potatoes and sweet potatoes, rice, pasta, breakfast cereals, dishes made from cereals such as maize, millet, oats and wheat, as well as plantains and green bananas. Most of us in this country currently get only a little over a quarter of our calorie intake this way.

Wholemeal bread and cereals are better than white or refined because they contain more vitamins, minerals, essential fatty acids and fibre, although most white bread also has added vitamins and minerals. But eating plenty, whether white, brown or wholemeal, is more important than insisting on wholemeal only. Carbohydrates have an undeserved reputation for causing weight gain. The blame really lies with the high-fat spreads and sauces we tend to accompany them with. Ounce for ounce, fat has twice the calories of carbohydrates.

Fibre

COMA recommends that the average person should aim for around 18g of fibre a day, with a maximum of 24g for big eaters and perhaps as little as 12g for small ones, measured by the New Englyst method. (The equivalent figures under the older Southgate method, which you may still see used on some labels, are 20g to 40g with an average of 30g. However, the Government favours the New Englyst method, and most big manufacturers and supermarkets are now using it.) To give you an idea what that means, 100g (3½oz) of wholemeal bread would contribute 9g to your diet, while the same weight of baked beans in tomato sauce would be 7.3g and of apple 2g.

Getting fibre just by adding raw bran to food is not as good as eating fibre-rich wholemeal foods. Uncooked bran contains phytates, which inhibit absorption of minerals like iron and zinc from food. Wholemeal foods are rich in fibre. Eating plenty of peas, beans and lentils is beneficial, too. Whole fruit and vegetables are better than juices because, as well as vitamins and other nutrients, they also contribute fibre to our diets.

Fat

COMA recommends that total fat intake should not exceed one-third of our daily calories. That is an average maximum of 90g for men and 70g for women, and means we need to cut our current average intake by about a sixth. Saturates (defined below), says COMA, need to be reduced even more drastically, to no more than 10 per cent, an average reduction of one-third.

The good news is that the more we fill up on carbohydrates, the more likely we are to avoid more fat-laden options such as some red meat, meat products and fatty snacks. It also helps if we choose lean-looking meat and leave the fat from meat and the skin from chicken on our plates. Meat products like pies, burgers and sauces often conceal high fat levels, as do cakes and biscuits.

If that seems tough, some experts believe the COMA figures are still too generous and would like to see the recommended limits for the intake of fats in total, and saturates in particular, set even lower. (However, people who are frail, very thin or with very poor appetites may need the more concentrated calories provided by food higher in fat.)

Salt

The WHO recommends that we restrict our salt intake to no more than 6g a day. That's less than half the 13g (two-and-a-half teaspoons) a day we now have on average. Most of us would probably deny we are having anything like this amount, but two-thirds of it is 'hidden' in manufactured foods. About half the rest occurs naturally in foods and the other half is added in cooking or at the table.

Protein

COMA says we can let the protein take care of itself. As we get older, our body's ability to digest and absorb protein decreases, so we need slightly more than we did when we were younger. Most people who live in the West get more than enough at every age.

To summarise

The message is simple:

- Eat as much fruit and vegetables as you like.
- Satisfy your appetite with starchy foods like bread, noodles and cereals (but be careful of adding fatty or sugary spreads or sauces).
- Watch carefully your intake of meat, fish and dairy products.

The ingredients

Carbohydrates

Plants make carbohydrates – starches and sugars – from carbon dioxide and water with the help of sunlight. All carbohydrates have the same basic ingredients – carbon, hydrogen and oxygen – but different carbohydrates combine them in different ways. Starches, or complex carbohydrates, consist of chains of glucose linked together, while sugars are more chemically straightforward. Complex carbohydrates are digested and broken down to simple carbohydrates over time – so keeping blood sugar levels on an even keel.

Carbohydrates are comparatively inexpensive and are a good source of other nutrients. For example, pulses, nuts and seeds provide carbohydrates, protein and vitamins E and B. (For more about vitamins, see below.)

Sugar

Sugar provides energy but no other nutrients at all: hence its reputation for being 'empty calories'. (A calorie is a measure of the energy that food can be converted into.) If our overall calorie intake is more than we need, sugar is of no benefit whatsoever.

Avoiding sugar in foods such as cakes, chocolate and biscuits makes a double contribution to healthy eating and weight control, because it includes cutting down on fat at the same time. Sugar gets the thumbs-down from dentists, too. It feeds the acid-producing bacteria that damage the surface of teeth and eventually wear through the enamel, causing tooth decay. Dental disease is actually the most widespread nutrition-related condition in Britain today.

Unfortunately, the British have a notorious sweet tooth. We get through an average of around 33kg (84lb) of sugar a year each. About half of it comes as hidden sugar in sweets, cakes, soft drinks and convenience foods.

Fibre

Fibre is the indigestible carbohydrate from plants. We need it to maintain a healthy digestive system. All fibre passes into the large intestine relatively unchanged. If it is soluble fibre, it dissolves in water there and forms a gooey liquid or gel and is fermented by bacteria. If it is insoluble, or what we used to call roughage, it passes out from the body basically unchanged.

Enough fibre helps prevent constipation in the short term and may also help prevent disorders of the intestine in the longer term. It seems from research that soluble fibre in oat bran (and, though not to the same extent, in pulses and lentils) can help bring down high cholesterol levels (see more about cholesterol below). Fibre also helps prevent diverticular disease, caused when small pouches develop in the wall of the large intestine and become infected and inflamed. Moreover, a high-fibre diet is sometimes successful in treating irritable bowel syndrome.

Fibre usually helps if you are trying to lose weight because the amount of chewing it requires imposes its own 'rationing system' on you – i.e. it takes relatively longer to eat high-fibre foods than low-fibre foods with the same number of calories – and because fibre helps meals feel satisfying by increasing their bulk without a corresponding increase in calories. Fibre may also inhibit the absorption of fats into the digestive system. Getting the full benefit of fibre depends on drinking enough (non-alcoholic) liquid. We need about a litre, or six to eight glasses, a day.

Fats

Fats are compounds of glycerol or common glycerine and fatty acids. So is cholesterol (see below). Fats can be **saturates**, **monounsaturates** or **polyunsaturates**. A fatty-acid molecule is made up of carbon and hydrogen atoms, and when the molecule is no longer capable of chemically receiving more hydrogen, the fat is termed 'saturated'. The molecules of unsaturated fats – mono-unsaturates or polyunsaturates – can take up more hydrogen in a chemical reaction.

Oils are 100 per cent fat and all have the same calorie content – about 135 calories a tablespoon. So anyone worrying about weight would want to keep his or her total fat intake down on those grounds alone. In addition, the total amount of oil in our diet also plays a role in determining our risk of heart disease and some cancers. But that is not the whole story.

Even more important in protecting oneself against heart disease than the total amount of fat we eat is our intake of saturates, the fats found mostly in foods of animal origin such as butter and cream, but also in coconut and palm oils. But that does not mean 'anything goes' when it comes to unsaturates.

Although polyunsaturates cut the risk of heart disease by reducing levels of harmful low-density lipoproteins, recent research suggests that too much polyunsaturated fat may also reduce the levels of beneficial high-density lipoproteins at the same time (see pp.85–7 for explanation of low- and high-density lipoproteins). Other experts interpret the findings to date as applying only to amounts of polyunsaturates that are so high they are unlikely to be found in a normal diet. The jury is still out on this one. On the other hand, monounsaturates, such as the fat contained in olive oil, have had a clean bill of health from research, including studies of the cholesterol and heart-disease levels of people living in Mediterranean countries, where olive oil is an important part of the daily diet.

So while research continues, the best advice at the moment seems to be to follow the universally accepted health education message to cut overall intake and to replace saturates as far as possible with a mixture of monounsaturates and polyunsaturates.

As a very rough guide, saturates are solid at room temperature and unsaturates are liquid, but it is not quite that simple. The process of industrial hardening of fats uses hydrogenation (a reaction between hydrogen and a metal catalyst) to convert unsaturates into saturates or into trans-saturated fatty acids, which behave like saturates in our bodies. You are unlikely to see 'trans-saturated fatty acids' listed on food labels. The clue to look for is the word 'hydrogenated'. The fats and oils in foods are often a mixture of saturates and unsaturates, in different proportions. Thus if you see a slogan such as 'high in polyunsaturates', you will still need to read the detailed contents breakdown to see the total amount of fat and just what proportion of it is which.

In some parts of the world, saturates account for as little as 3 per cent of the calories in the local diet. We don't actually need any at all. In the UK, about 17 per cent of our energy on average comes from saturates, and in Scotland, where men have the worst rates of heart disease in the world, it reaches 20 per cent, almost double the healthy intake.

Essential fatty acids

Essential fatty acids belong to two groups. They are termed 'essential' because they are vital for life and we cannot make them ourselves. The omega-6 family comes from vegetable oils like sunflower, and omega-3 comes from some vegetable oils such as soya-bean and rapeseed oils, and from oily fish.

There is now evidence that an intake of more than a bare minimum of omega-3 fatty acids may protect us against heart and other disease. Fish that are rich in omega-3 fatty acids include salmon, mackerel, sardines, pilchards, herrings, kippers and fresh or frozen tuna (not canned – the canning process used for tuna destroys fatty acids). Making a point of having oily fish at least once a week is good health insurance.

Protein

Proteins consist of large molecules made up from smaller units called amino acids. The digestive system breaks protein down into its constituent amino acids to use them as it needs in order to synthesise new proteins for its own growth and for tissue repair, and to make chemical messengers like adrenaline, enzymes for digestion, and antibodies to ward off infection.

Protein manufacture is a bit like stringing different-coloured beads in a pre-determined pattern on a thread. But if the body does not have exactly the amino acids it wants, it stops stringing altogether. It has a limited ability to convert one into another, and some cannot be made in the body at all. If we don't get enough of them directly from our diet, we go without, although this isn't usually a problem in the West.

Protein from sources such as pulses, lentils, brown rice and wholemeal grains is cheaper than protein from meat and is also lower in fat and richer in dietary fibre.

Salt

Some salt is essential for us. But we eat, on average, about two-and-a-half teaspoons of salt a day, slightly more than twice the maximum the WHO says we should. Much of our current average intake comes from salt added to manufactured foods, and we add about half the rest in cooking or at the table. Some is naturally present in foods. (Expect to find 'sodium' rather than 'salt' on some food labels; 2300mg of sodium is equivalent to about 6g of salt, which is about what we should aim not to exceed in a day.) Reducing your salt intake may lower your blood pressure.

Vitamins

Vitamins are chemically unrelated to one another. They are all organic substances we need to get in small amounts from our diet because our bodies are unable to manufacture them either at all or in sufficient quantities.

They are needed for growth and repair of tissues, growth and maintenance of healthy skin, good vision and strong teeth and bones. Unlike proteins, carbohydrates and fats, vitamins don't supply energy to the body, but some are needed to enable energy to be released from other foods.

More vitamins probably remain to be discovered, and there is much we do not yet understand about those that are known. Their names have no significance beyond the order in which they were discovered.

Vitamins are divided into two groups. The **water-soluble** B vitamins and vitamin C are easily lost in cooking (simply because they do dissolve in water), though some can be salvaged – for example, by using vegetable cooking water to make gravy. The body does not store significant quantities of them, so we need some in our diet every day. **Fat-soluble** vitamins A, D, E and K are stored in the liver, and a good intake of them about once a week is usually enough. An extremely good source of vitamin A is liver; in fact, a single portion will provide enough for a month (though liver is not recommended if you are pregnant).

There has been considerable excitement in nutritional circles in recent years about the antioxidants beta–carotene, a precursor of vitamin A, and vitamins C and E, plus the mineral selenium. They apparently offer some protection from illnesses, particularly cancers and heart disease. Their role seems to be that they prevent fat from going rancid in the body by mopping up free radicals of oxygen. Free radicals are unstable molecules that seem to damage our cells as they try to replace electrons missing from their own structures by stealing them from other molecules. Many researchers are now convinced that it is such cell damage that has a role in triggering heart disease and cancers. Antioxidants seem to be able to give electrons to free radicals to complete their structures for them, without themselves becoming unstable and thus having to go electron-raiding themselves.

Fruit and vegetables provide one of the best sources of the antioxidants, and eating plenty of them does seem to protect us against heart disease and some cancers. Research has yet to discover whether the beneficial effect is caused by the presence of antioxidants themselves, or something else in fruit and vegetables, or by a combination of the two. The Government has funded a three-year research programme to find out more about antioxidants, and the World Health Organization decided at the end of 1992 there was enough evidence to justify a large-scale trial. But whatever underlying mechanism or mechanisms are eventually discovered to explain the benefits, the healthy-eating message will remain the same: lots of fruit and vegetables are a major contribution to a healthy diet.

Vitamin supplements

People who follow the COMA and WHO guidelines above and have a varied diet – one that includes complex carbohydrates, dairy products, fruit and vegetables, rice and grains, and protein sources such as meat, poultry, fish and pulses – usually don't need vitamin supplements.

At best, taking supplements unnecessarily is a waste of money. At worst, it can be harmful. Overdosing on water-soluble vitamins can cause unpleasant side effects such as nausea and vomiting, although – except for B6 – the excess can be excreted in urine and does not accumulate in the body. More serious is too high an intake of the fat-soluble vitamins, which do accumulate. People have actually died from too much vitamin A. An overdose of vitamin C can destroy precious B12; iron and zinc are also poisonous in excess.

Some people are more at risk of vitamin deficiency than others. They include:

- People unwilling or unable to prepare nutritious meals for themselves, especially if they are living alone or have poor appetites.

- Smokers, who have lower levels of antioxidants in their blood than non-smokers and may benefit from a higher intake of the A, C and E vitamins plus selenium.
- Vegetarians, especially if they are vegan, who need to be careful that they get enough vitamin D and calcium. They need to be careful, too, about getting enough vitamin B12, either by eating foods supplemented with it (such as spreads containing yeast extracts, certain kinds of soya milks and some breakfast cereals), or by taking a supplement directly.
- Elderly people and those on long-term drug treatment, who may not absorb vitamins well and may run short of some of the B vitamins and vitamin C. Illness also depletes vitamin C, which cannot be stored in the body.
- People who do not take milk or dairy foods, who thus might not be getting enough calcium. (See also under Brittle bones, below.)
- Crash or long-term dieters.

In a one-year study done in Newfoundland and reported in *The Lancet* (7 November 1992), volunteers over the age of 65 were given extra vitamins and had their immune systems boosted (as shown by laboratory tests). They had fewer days of illness (7, compared with 23) than those on the placebo. But all 96 volunteers had vitamin deficiencies at the start. The results leave open the question of whether such deficiencies are better addressed by improvement in diet or by taking vitamin supplements.

Certainly, for most of us, getting the vitamins and minerals we need from real food is preferable to taking supplements. This is true not only because it is cheaper to do so, but also because food gives us other important things our body needs, such as fibre. A healthy diet which follows the COMA/WHO guidelines will give us the minerals and vitamins we need. But the answer is not so clear-cut for people at special nutritional risk (such as the groups outlined above).

Minerals and trace elements

As well as carbohydrates, proteins and fats, which are all compounds containing the element carbon, we also need some minerals in their inorganic form – i.e. not bound to carbon. The

Table 1: VITAMINS AND MINERALS

Vitamins & minerals	Function in body	Main sources	How lost
A	Growth, night vision, healthy skin	Liver, green leafy veg, carrots, eggs, cheese, milk	Exposure to light and air, cooking in hot fats
B1: thiamine	Release of energy from foods	Potatoes, wholemeal and white bread, veg, milk, breakfast cereals, pulses, nuts	Cooking, especially with bicarbonate of soda or baking soda
B2: riboflavin	Release of energy from foods	Liver, meat, milk and cheese	Exposure to light
B3: niacin or nicotinic acid	Release of energy from foods	Pulses, liver, meat, bread, cereal	Leaching into cooking fluids (not destroyed, can be reused)
B5: pantothenic acid	Energy production	Liver, kidney, eggs, peanuts, mushrooms, cheese, pears	Dissolving in cooking water; also heat, freezing, milling, canning, contact with bicarbonate of soda
B6: pyridoxine	Metabolism of proteins	Liver, cereals, pulses, poultry	Leaching into cooking water; destroyed by light
B12: cobalamin	Formation of red blood cells	Meat, milk, cheese, eggs	Contact with bicarbonate of soda in cooking water
B: folic acid	Formation of red blood cells	Green leafy veg	Heat, air and long or poor storage; also leached into cooking liquids

B: biotin	Energy production from fat	Liver, pork, kidneys, nuts, cauliflower, lentils, cereals	Cooking, especially with bicarbonate of soda or baking soda
C: ascorbic acid	Healing wounds, aids iron absorption	Citrus fruits, blackcurrants, green leafy veg, potatoes, tomatoes	Light, air, time, bruising, soaking, contact with bicarbonate of soda, use of copper pots
D	Helps body use calcium for healthy bones and teeth	Sunlight, margarine, fatty fish, eggs, butter	Little; it is remarkably stable
E	Protects against harmful substances in your blood	Vegetable oils, nuts, eggs, butter, wholegrain cereals	When oils are heated, in refining and processing, even during storage in refrigerator or freezer
K	Nature's 'bandaid' which prevents bleeding	Many, especially vegetables and dairy products	Not easily
Calcium	Builds bones and teeth	Milk, cheese, sardines, yogurt	In refining, and not taken up without enough vitamin D; raw bran also interferes with uptake
Iron	Prevents anaemia	Red meat, liver, beans, dried fruit, nuts, bread	In refining and processing; absorption inhibited by phytic acid in cereals and pulses, tannin in tea and coffee
Zinc	Helps cells to divide and grow	Meat, liver, herring, milk, turkey, wholegrain foods	By refining; absorption slows as we age

Most people get all the vitamins and minerals they need from a healthy diet; they don't need to take supplements.

convention is that the ones of which we need more than 100mg a day – including calcium, magnesium and sodium – are called minerals, and those of which we need less – such as iron, iodine, zinc and selenium – are called trace elements.

The essential minerals make up about 1 per cent of our diet and are important for water balance, skeleton development and blood production. Getting enough of them is as important as making sure we do not get too much sodium and chloride (which is why we need to keep down our intake of salt). Actually, people who have dietary problems because they are eating too little or not eating a balanced enough diet, or who are on drugs that interfere with nutrition (for example diuretics), are more likely to be deficient in trace elements or minerals than they are in vitamins.

Selenium

This trace element has come in for its share of attention as one of the antioxidants (along with beta-carotene – the precursor of vitamin A – and vitamins C and E) mentioned above. Although it seems to have a role in protecting against heart disease and some cancers, it is still comparatively recently discovered and little understood. We know we need only small amounts of it, but not yet exactly how small, although nutritionists tend to support a figure between 25 and 70 millionths of a gram a day. Moreover, it is difficult to calculate how much we are getting, because the same type of food grown or raised in different places with different soils can vary in selenium content. It is found in meat, especially kidney, and in brazil nuts, oily fish, bread and rice, and lost in processing and refining.

Magnesium

Essential for many of the chemical processes that keep our body's cells working, magnesium helps break down food for energy, build bones and improve the absorption of calcium (see below) and of vitamin B6. Important though magnesium is, getting enough of it is unlikely to be a problem for most people. Our bodies are very efficient at regulating their own magnesium content, and the mineral is in a wide variety of foods and in tap water.

Zinc

Because zinc is needed for growth and repair, it has a role in healing. It is also essential for taste and flavour perception. Zinc is found in meat and poultry, fish and seafood, milk, yogurt, cottage cheese, beans, pulses and wholegrain foods.

Iron

Iron comes in two forms. Haem is from animal sources and is efficiently absorbed, and non-haem is from vegetable and grain foods and is less well taken up, although it does better if there is vitamin C present. Some evidence seems to suggest that tea and coffee may decrease absorption. Iron makes haemoglobin, which gives red blood cells their colour and transports oxygen around the body. We need iron to prevent anaemia, which causes tiredness, lack of stamina and even reduced brain function. It is found in red meat, kidney and liver, poultry, seafood, fish (including canned tuna), cereals, chocolate, nuts and wholemeal bread.

Calcium

Calcium is of enormous importance in building and maintaining a healthy body, helping the blood to clot, ensuring normal heart function and helping control cholesterol levels (see below). It also helps the body absorb vitamin B12. Milk and milk products, including yogurt, are good sources. So are sardines, whitebait, tofu, watercress, parsley, dried figs, nuts (especially almonds), soya flour, dried apricots, cabbage, oatmeal and sesame seeds. Mass-manufactured white bread also has calcium added, and some tap waters contain a lot.

Brittle bones Most of the calcium in our bodies, 98 per cent of it, is used in our bones, while 1 per cent is in our teeth and the remaining 1 per cent circulates in the blood. Calcium is constantly moving in and out of our bones, and when the level in our blood falls too low, it takes the calcium out of the bones to top it up. If this keeps happening, the bones become weaker.

Loss of calcium leads to osteoporosis, or the thinning of bones, which leaves them weak and porous and more easily broken. It affects women more than men, for a number of reasons. Among them are that, after the menopause, women no longer manufacture the hormone oestrogen, which, it seems, has a protective effect on bones. Adding to the problem is the fact that many middle-aged women have histories of avoiding calcium-rich dairy foods through years of dieting.

Some authorities now believe that as men, too, begin to live longer they will increasingly suffer the same condition. It will just come later for them. Adequate calcium intake right through life is the first line of defence against osteoporosis, and dairy products – especially skimmed milk because it is low in fat – are an ideal source.

Some experts believe that eating more calcium has no impact on the rapid rate of bone loss at the menopause, except when calcium intakes are very low. Others disagree and insist that large intakes of calcium can reduce bone loss. The daily amount of calcium recommended by the Government for adults is currently 700mg. But recent research from New Zealand and France published in the *New England Journal of Medicine* suggests that post-menopausal women need 1000mg. The National Osteoporosis Society is now advising women over 45 to make sure they have 1500mg a day, or 1000mg if they are on hormone replacement therapy (HRT).

CHANGES IN BONE MASS

The curves represent an average, but individual bone mass varies a lot. Nobody has traced bone mass for a lifetime using modern bone measurement techniques, but the curves give a general picture of the changes thought to take place.

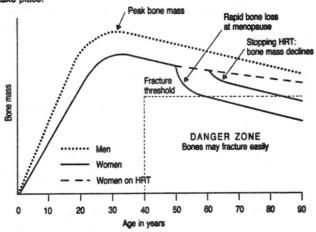

A pint of full-cream, semi-skimmed or skimmed milk provides about 750mg. There are also milks on the market that have been specially calcium-enriched, and dried skimmed-milk powder can be added as an extra to dishes. Canned sardines, cottage cheese and low-fat yogurt are also good healthy sources.

Women on hormone replacement therapy (discussed further in Chapter 5) not only protect their bones from calcium loss while they are on it, but also seem to enjoy a bone-loss slow-down for a time even after they stop.

Smoking, lack of exercise, a diet high in fat or protein or containing phytates (found in raw bran), and ageing all also interfere with calcium uptake and encourage calcium loss.

Making the recipe work

Here are some ways you might think about starting to put the guidelines for healthy eating into practice with a minimum of disruption – and pain:

Shopping

- Look for lower fat or reduced-fat versions of favourite foods in the supermarket and try them out. Don't be deceived by slogans. 'Light' or 'lite' can have many meanings, so be sure to read the small print.
- Labels like 'lean' and 'extra-lean' can mean different things in different supermarkets, too. Again, check the details on the label.
- Don't just note the figure for 'sugar' on labels. Fructose, sucrose, dextrose, glucose, maltose, honey, syrup, raw sugar, cane sugar, muscovado sugar and concentrated fruit juice all mean sugar, too.
- Try to cut back, gradually if it hurts, on how much jam, marmalade, syrup, treacle and honey you buy.
- Cut down on salt by flavouring more with herbs, lemon juice and so on. Use lower-salt and lower-sugar versions of baked beans and other tinned foods.
- Check the small print on ready-made breakfast cereals and snacks and try to avoid the ones with coconut or palm oil in them.

- Switch to semi-skimmed or, especially if being overweight is a problem, skimmed milk.
- Switch from butter to a spread that is lower in saturates (or just spread your butter thinner).
- Be aware that most cooking oils (coconut is an exception) are lower in saturates than are butter, lard and other traditional solid fats.

Food preparation

- Grill rather than fry.
- If you do fry, try stir-frying. The technique is to use a hot wok (or frying pan) and a tiny amount of oil. You need to have everything prepared in advance and keep it all moving fast as it cooks. Start with what will need the most cooking and add ingredients in order of cooking time. This can make a little meat or seafood go a long way, and give leftovers a new lease of life.
- When roasting, prick the skin of duck, goose and turkey so that fat is shed during cooking. (A tin of water under a turkey and a foil cover on top stops it drying out too much as a result.)
- Take as much fat as you can from the roasting pan before you make the gravy.
- Use one of those gravy boats with two spouts and use the one that pours from below the surface. (Fat settles on the top and can be poured off through the other.)
- If you can, make stock, casseroles and so forth ahead of time, and chill to solidify fat on top so you can remove it. (Flavours will mingle better, too, if you do.)
- Most recipes don't need the ingredients browned in fat at the start. They work just as well if you put everything in the pot together cold.
- But if you are browning, do it in fat hot enough to seal the surfaces. (If it's not hot enough, it will soak into the food.) Brown a little at a time so fat temperature does not drop too much, and drain off as much fat as you can before you go on to the next stage.
- Most recipes work well with much less oil/fat than they say. (Generally, the older the cookery book, the more you can get away with reducing it.)

- Cook vegetables in as little unsalted water as you can to mini-mise vitamin loss. And use any water left over in gravy, stock or sauces.
- Conserve nutritional value by not preparing vegetables ahead of time or pre-soaking; this will prevent loss of vitamins B and C in the water.
- Remember that the smaller you cut or shred vegetables, the more vitamins you are likely to lose.
- In recipes that call for cream, use instead evaporated skimmed milk, buttermilk or low-fat yogurt.
- Don't leave milk on the doorstep. It loses valuable vitamin B2 if you do.
- Low-fat or almost fat-free fromage frais, with its lovely creamy texture, works just as well with sweet or savoury flavourings. (If you use it instead of cream in sauces, add it off the heat to prevent curdling.)
- Serve food as soon as you can after cooking.

Menus

- If your main meals tend to fall into the meat/fish-and-two-veg category, start experimenting with pasta, pulses and rice dishes some days.
- Another way to cut the quantity of meat at a meal is to use noodles or pasta on the side to make it all the more filling.
- Beans, pulses and grains are almost fat-free. Serve them along-side reduced meat portions, or go all the way and serve them instead.
- Try routinely halving your meat portions and doubling the vegetables.
- Avoid meat products such as sausages, luncheon meats, pies. They tend to be higher in fat than lean meat alone.
- Ditto processed chicken products such as chicken pies.
- If you are using highly spiced flavourings with mince, use lower-fat turkey instead of beef.
- Oven chips have less fat than deep-fried ones, and large-cut deep-fried chips have less than thin-cut.
- Go for fish, which is low in fat, in preference to red meat, at least some of the time.

- Chicken has less fat if you don't eat the skin. Turkey has less still.
- Venison has less than a third of the fat of beef.
- Salad is good for us; salad dressing often isn't. Make a dressing with olive oil, which is monounsaturated, if you don't have a weight problem. If you do, experiment with commercial low-fat versions or make your own based on yogurt, fromage frais, tomato juice or liquidised tofu.
- Check out reduced-fat cheeses. Or go the other route and use the strongest-flavoured cheese you can find for sauces and so on so that you will need less.
- Try to replace cakes, biscuits and pastries as snacks with fruit, crispbreads, rice cakes and even dried fruit.
- Never say never about your favourite foods. No matter how unhealthy something is, it is a sounder psychological tactic to allow yourself to have it as an occasional treat than to tell yourself you may never have it again.

There are many more shopping, cooking and menu planning hints and more detailed nutritional information in the Which? Consumer Guide *Which? Way to a Healthier Diet*★★.

Troubleshooting

There are two further essential ingredients of a healthy diet, and that is understanding how to deal positively and constructively with two of the most widespread health bug-bears of being 40-plus: high cholesterol and weight control.

Cholesterol

Cholesterol is a waxy alcohol essential in forming all animal-cell membranes and needed for proper nerve function. It is also essential for a number of other vital processes, including the manufacture of vitamin D and of hormones, particularly those regulating metabolism, and digestion. It is actually a soft, white, odourless powder that does not mix with water.

We don't need any cholesterol at all in our diets. The body makes all the cholesterol it needs, mainly in the liver. Too much does us no good at all. The deposits of fatty plaque that clog coronary arteries and cause heart attacks and strokes consist mainly of cholesterol.

The story is not a simple one. Because cholesterol doesn't mix with water, it can travel through the blood only if it is attached to water-soluble substances. Three proteins, called lipoproteins, perform this function. (Lipo means fat.)

Two of them – **low-density lipoprotein (LDL)** and **very-low-density lipoprotein (VLDL)** – carry cholesterol to the linings of blood vessels. They are involved in the development of atherosclerosis, or hardening of the arteries, which can lead to coronary heart disease or strokes by reducing the blood supply to the heart or brain. LDL particles become oxidised and then taken up by blood cells called monocytes. It is these monocytes, engorged with LDL-cholesterol, that become lodged in the artery walls, gradually making the artery channel narrower.

The accumulation of plaque on blood vessel walls not only narrows them and so restricts the flow of blood to tissues but also enables clots to attach to the walls more easily. The narrower the blood vessel, the more likely it is that a clot will cause a blockage. When deposits of fatty streaks build up into hard fibrous lumps (like bad porridge) big enough to block an artery, they cause a heart attack or a stroke, depending on which artery they are blocking. VLDL also carries blood triglycerides, or fats, high levels of which make the blood more likely to clot. Studies have shown that lowering the LDL level in our blood can slow atherosclerosis and sometimes even reverse its effects.

The third lipoprotein, **high-density lipoprotein (HDL)**, carries cholesterol away from the vessel walls and is called 'good' cholesterol because it seems to have the effect of protecting against atherosclerosis. HDL levels are increased by exercise, a vegetarian diet and, for post-menopausal women, hormone replacement therapy.

Besides the cholesterol we manufacture for ourselves, there is more in almost all food of animal origin. The highest concentration is in egg yolk, fish roe and offal such as liver, kidney and brain. Cholesterol is virtually absent from food of vegetable origin.

The relationship between dietary and blood cholesterol is not a simple one, either. Generally, the more we eat, the less our bodies produce, which for many of us helps keep blood cholesterol at a tolerable level. One person in two in Britain has high blood cholesterol. But for one person in five this feedback mechanism does not work at all efficiently and their level is very high.

An even more important determinant of blood cholesterol than dietary cholesterol for these people is the effect of total fat consumption in general, and especially of saturates. The underlying mechanism is believed to be that high levels of LDL and cholesterol are caused by a defect in the receptor that has the job of removing LDL from the blood. A diet high in saturates seems to make this receptor even less efficient, thus exacerbating the problem.

High blood cholesterol is only one of the risk factors of coronary heart disease, but keeping it under control will reduce the danger. People with a family or personal history that suggests higher-than-average risk – including survivors of heart attacks and bypass surgery – may be advised by their doctors to stick to an even lower total- and saturated-fat intake than the guidelines recommend for the rest of us.

High cholesterol levels in the blood sometimes leave clues on the surface of the body. If you are under 50 and can see a white circle around the edge of your iris (the coloured part of the eye), it could be a sign of a high cholesterol level. So could small fatty lumps on the eyelids or on the tendons at the back of the ankles or wrists. But the only way to find out for sure is to have your blood cholesterol level tested.

If you want a test, go to your doctor. It is better to have it as part of an assessment of all your heart-disease-risk factors than to use a DIY kit or have a test done in a health shop or pharmacy. Besides, when *Which? way to Health* magazine assessed home testing kits (results published in the February 1993 issue), the results were variable. In one case, a man in his 60s had readings as low as 5.78 and as high as 7.8 with three different testing kits used the same day.

The test will be done on a blood sample either from your arm or from a finger prick. Don't use hand cream beforehand: if the cream contains cholesterol, it may interfere with the result.

Some tests give a breakdown of LDL and HDL cholesterol, and others give only the total of blood cholesterol, which is generally enough to be a good indicator of harmful LDL, as the table below explains:

Table 2: WHAT THE TEST RESULTS MEAN

Cholesterol level	Risk of heart disease
Less than 5.2	Low
5.2–6.5	Some increased risk
6.5–7.8	Moderate risk
Over 7.8	High risk

If your reading is 6.5, you have twice the risk of developing heart disease that someone with a reading of 5.2 has (assuming your other risk factors are equal).

There is evidence that:

- Cutting your total intake of fat even to the 30 per cent of calories or less recommended in the COMA guidelines (see above) can reduce blood cholesterol levels by about 10 per cent, which translates into a 20 per cent reduction of the risk of heart disease.
- People monitored on a low-fat diet had large enough reductions in artery blockage to show up on an X-ray. They also had fewer new blockages than a control group that had not switched to a low-fat diet.

Your weight: How much is too much?

We gain weight when we are getting more energy from our food than we are using up in our daily lives, and our bodies are storing the excess as fat. The solution involves both sides of the energy equation: we need to be sure that we are exercising enough (as discussed in the previous two chapters) and that we are not eating too many calories.

Most people who have had a yo-yo weight problem throughout their 20s and 30s find it doesn't get any easier in their 40s and 50s. Even people who always once seemed to be able to eat what they liked and get away with it can find the scales starting to creep up on them somewhere after 40.

The impact on your health of being overweight depends on two things: how much excess weight there is and where it has settled.

Obesity is the *excessive* accumulation of body fat, excessive enough to put health at risk. It is not just being a little on the plump side of what we would like to see looking back at us in the mirror. Obesity is gauged by the body mass index (BMI), which isn't a direct measurement of fat but gives a good working indication of fat status.

To find out your BMI, divide your weight in kilograms by the square of your height in metres. So, for example, if you are 5ft 4ins (1.63 metres) and weigh 9st 9lb (61kg), you multiply 1.63 x 1.63 which gives 2.66, and divide 61 by 2.66 to give 23, which is below the 25 threshold for even slight obesity.

If you score between 20 and 25, you are at a lower risk of heart disease and a number of other health threats. If you score between 25 and 29.9, you are rated slightly fat and the risk is starting to rise. From 30 to 40, your rating is moderately obese, and from 40 upwards, you are really taking chances with your health. Underweight is undesirable for good health, too. A BMI of under 20 means there can be increased risk of a number of problems, including depression and osteoporosis. The chart below gives you a quick check of whether you are a healthy weight.

ARE YOU THE RIGHT WEIGHT?

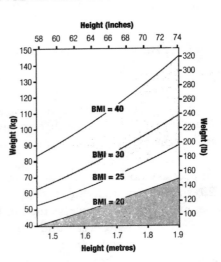

Use this chart to check your 'body mass index' (BMI) or whether you're the right weight for your height. If your BMI score is below 20, you are under-weight; 20–25 is ideal; 25–30 means you are overweight; and 30+ means you are seriously overweight – see your doctor

Research now suggests it is not just a matter of how much excess weight you wear, but where you wear it. There seems to be an 'apples and pears' relationship between excess weight and resulting risk. Being overweight poses a bigger health threat, it seems, if you carry most of your excess around your waist — in the apple shape many chubby men have. If your excess comes to roost more on your hips, in the pear shape more usual for overweight women, the risk is lower. Genetics determines whether you are an 'apple' or a 'pear', but you are taking a bigger gamble with your health if you are an 'apple' and don't watch your weight.

Scientists in Sweden have been using the results of this research to design experiments giving men doses of the male hormone testosterone in a stick-on stomach patch. The patch does not make the fat disappear, they say, but shifts it to other parts of the body where it poses less of a threat to health.

The average beer-lover's 'gut' is trimmed by an inch by this method, a 'significant amount', according to Dr George Bray, editor of the American magazine *Obesity Research*, which published the findings. The patch — planned for sale in the US and Europe if further tests prove positive — has the reported side effect of boosting the sex drive of the experimental subjects. Meanwhile, a reduction in beer intake promises to shift unwanted waistline inches not to another part of the anatomy, but off the body altogether. And it is not the only way to lose weight.

For successful slimming, remember that:

- Slowly does it. Aim for a maximum loss of 2lb (approximately 1kg) a week, and 1lb each week is better after the first week or two. (You may lose more the first couple of weeks because part of what you are shedding is water.) Weight that comes off fast usually goes back fast. Worse, if you are losing fast, you may be losing lean tissue rather than fat. Eventually that will slow down the rate at which you burn calories, so you will gain weight more easily than before. With serious starvation diets, you can even lose organ tissue such as heart muscle.

- Avoid 'dieting' in the sense of trying to eat sparingly according to rigid rules over a set period of time. Long-term success lies in adopting a healthy eating pattern for life, not 'going on a diet'.

- The general rules are the same as for healthy eating at any weight — lots of fruit and vegetables, watch the fat and sugar, fill up on complex carbohydrates such as bread and pasta (without lashings of butter or creamy sauces), and keep portions of meat, poultry and fish small.

- Adopt as many of the tips described on pp.81–4 as you can for reducing the fat and sugar content of your diet. The more you do, the more easily you will get the fat off.

- Eating 'real food' is a far better way to slim than using commercial slimming products. It leads to long-term good eating habits. When *Which?* magazine investigated slimming plans (reported July 1993), it found that the 13 meal replacements assessed were often high in fat, sugar and calories, and only one plan could show the researchers proof of long-term success. The conclusion: many diet foods help you lose £££s.

Herbal slimming patches on the market in the UK haven't been shown to help weight loss, and Department of Health tests found they contained so little of the active ingredient (claimed to be natural and herbal) that they were unlikely to have any effect. The Advertising Standards Authority has said newspapers and magazines should not accept advertisements for them.

There are no magic shortcuts to a healthy diet. But the pay-off of adopting such a diet can seem little short of magical in its effects.

CHAPTER 4

SMOKING AND DRINKING

WHETHER we smoke and what and how much we drink are important in determining how fit and healthy we are in the 40-plus years. For smoking, the health message is clear – don't. Giving up does us more good than any other single life-style change we can make.

When it comes to what and how much we drink, the story is more ambiguous. For alcohol, on the negative side are the facts that the combination of drinking and driving is often a killer on the roads and, even if we keep our drinking and driving apart, too much alcohol does our bodies no favours. It is by no means all bad news, however: recent studies show that perhaps a little of what we fancy may be good for us.

For coffee and tea drinkers, too, moderation is key. Research into possible links between excess coffee drinking and serious illness has so far – except in the case of boiled coffee – been inconclusive. It is clear, however, that some people would benefit from cutting out coffee altogether.

Smoking

The single most significant life-style change that anyone can make to improve his or her health dramatically is to give up smoking. The more we know about tobacco, the more damning the case against its use becomes.

Smoking is a risk at any age, but the longer we postpone a decision to quit, the more we are pushing our luck. Come 40, and we are chancing it. At 50, we are really starting to hit crunch time, if we are still smoking. Yet even at 60 and beyond, it still pays to give up.

The case against tobacco

A major study that began back in 1948 in the town of Framingham on the east coast of America has become a major source of information about coronary heart disease. It has found smokers two to three times as susceptible to heart problems as non-smokers. The British Regional Heart Study, which is watching the health of 8000 men aged between 40 and 50 in 24 towns in Britain, has come to similar conclusions.

Other recent research has looked not only at how much smoking increases the risk of heart disease but also at how much giving up smoking puts the risk clock back again. Several major studies which between them have followed the fortunes of more than 250,000 subjects over four decades have concluded that once people have been ex-smokers for long enough, the risks to their health are no longer much greater than those of people who have never smoked. For heart disease, some studies have found that after five years the risks are almost as low for ex-smokers as for non-smokers. Other research has concluded that this risk-lowering process takes 10 to 15 years. Similarly, the relative danger of lung cancer is only slightly greater for ex-smokers after 10 to 15 non-smoking years than it is for people who have never smoked.

But the important point is that there does not come a day when the slate is suddenly 'wiped clean' – allowing the former smoker to start life again with no more risk than if he or she had never smoked. There is a gradual improvement in health and a reduction in risk almost from the first smoke-free day; and that improvement is quickly eroded if an ex-smoker resumes the habit.

Carbon monoxide is a poisonous gas present in cigarette smoke which combines with haemoglobin, the oxygen–carrying substance in the blood, even more readily than oxygen does. As a result, 15 per cent of a smoker's blood may be carrying carbon monoxide instead of oxygen. As soon as a smoker gives up, the blood starts carrying more of the oxygen that is so essential for the efficient functioning of all tissues and body cells. And that is just the first benefit of many.

Smokers' capillaries (the smallest blood vessels) constrict under the influence of increased adrenaline and other substances produced when the stimulant nicotine prods the adrenal glands into stepping up production of them. Becoming an ex-smoker allows the capillaries to expand again, so blood can move more easily to the extremities, heart and brain.

Lung function is back to normal after three months without cigarettes, as long as lung structure had suffered no permanent damage before smoking was given up. After one year, the risk of coronary heart disease has dropped significantly.

Although the evidence of the dangers of smoking is undeniable, the picture is, of course, complicated. People may have a high risk of heart disease for other reasons. What the major studies have found is that adding smoking to other risk factors, such as high blood pressure and high levels of cholesterol, magnifies the danger enormously. An important factor in determining the odds of a heart attack is age – another reason to give up smoking now, rather than let the age-smoke combination multiply into a greater risk.

It used to be reckoned that of 1000 young people smoking 20 or more cigarettes a day in the UK, one would be murdered, six would die in road accidents and 250 would die prematurely as a result of their smoking. Recent research, however, suggests that 250 was an underestimate.

One study by Richard Peto, reported in *The Lancet* in 1992, estimated that one smoker in three dies of smoking-related diseases. Half of them die before they reach 70 – an average of 24 years earlier than they would have done had they not smoked – and the other half after 70, still eight years sooner than they otherwise would have done.

The catalogue of damage that tobacco does to smokers is a grim one, which includes:

- increasing the risk of sudden death
- making coronary heart disease more likely
- magnifying the threat of heart disease even more dramatically for people who are already at greater risk from high blood pressure or high blood cholesterol, or both
- doubling the chances of another heart attack for people who have already had one
- causing thickening and hardening of the arteries that supply the brain, which in turn could lead to a stroke

- damaging the arteries that supply the legs, which in some cases could lead to gangrene and amputation
- increasing the risk of emphysema, chronic bronchitis and asthma – and the frequency of attacks for people who have asthma
- boosting the risk of lung cancer
- being instrumental in causing cancers of the mouth, nose, throat, larynx, oesophagus, cervix, kidney, bladder and pancreas, and leukaemia
- damaging and reducing the efficiency of the lungs (an average non-smoker aged 75 will still have three-quarters of the useful lung capacity of his or her youth, while a smoker will have only about one quarter – a huge difference)
- augmenting the frequency of everyday complaints such as coughs, sneezes and shortness of breath on exertion
- increasing the danger of osteoporosis (loss of bone mass leading to increased danger of fractures) for post-menopausal women and bringing menopause forward by two to three years on average for women
- making the likelihood of getting a peptic ulcer greater, and making it more difficult for peptic ulcers to be healed
- interfering with the effectiveness of various medications
- decreasing energy – making you feel less fit
- ageing the skin, making it appear wrinkled and drier.

Passive smoking

The passive smoking which smokers inflict on non-smokers in the same room with them has two facets: it is both what the smoker has inhaled and exhaled again (called 'mainstream smoke') and the smoke that comes from the burning end of a cigarette or cigar sitting in an ashtray between puffs or from the tobacco smouldering in a pipe ('sidestream smoke').

Sidestream smoke may be worse than mainstream, since it has not gone through the double filtering system of the cigarette's filter and the smoker's lungs. Thus it may contain higher concentrations of dangerous chemicals. Passive smokers get about four times as much sidestream as mainstream smoke.

Avoiding being a passive smoker makes us much healthier. Inhaling other people's smoke makes us more likely to:

- die of lung cancer – long-term passive smoking increases the risk of getting lung cancer for non-smokers from 10 per cent to 30 per cent, according to recent research
- suffer damage to the heart, according to a recent review of 11 studies of the link between heart disease and passive smoking
- suffer irritation to eyes, nose and throat, and headaches and dizziness
- be more seriously affected if we have asthma or allergies.

Enormously affected are the children of smokers, who inhale the same amount of nicotine as if they themselves had smoked 60 to 150 cigarettes a year, according to a recent report published by the National Children's Bureau. Children of smokers are likely to:

- have higher rates of bronchitis, pneumonia and middle-ear infections
- be, on average, one centimetre shorter at primary-school age
- be, on average, up to six months behind their classmates in reading, maths and other subjects at the age of 11.

Although poverty and poor nutrition may also affect children's health, size and physical and mental development, smoking has a separate measurable effect. Women who smoke during pregnancy also tend to have smaller babies, and some of the differences outlined above may result not just from passive smoking throughout childhood but also from the mother's smoking during pregnancy.

What's in smoke?

Cigarette smoke is a cocktail of somewhere around 5000 different chemicals, some of which are known toxins (poisons) and others known carcinogens (cancer-causers). They include the following:

Nicotine This powerful stimulant prods the adrenal glands into secreting substances such as adrenaline in order to increase heart rate and blood pressure and constrict the capillaries, thus decreasing the amount of oxygen available to heart and brain. Although many smokers like to think that a cigarette helps them relax, smoking actually simulates stress, keeping the body in a state of heightened tension. In addition, the liver has to detoxify nicotine, and asking it to do too much of that can impair liver function, just as too much alcohol does.

Carbon monoxide Because smokers breathe in such a cocktail of chemicals, they take in less oxygen in the first place. On top of that, carbon monoxide displaces the oxygen carried by red blood cells, making what oxygen there is less available to the heart and other tissues, in turn forcing the heart to work harder. This is just one of the reasons why smokers run out of breath faster than do non-smokers.

Cyanide Hydrogen cyanide reduces the ability of the tiny cilia, the hairs that line the lungs, to clean out unwanted substances such as tars.

Tars Tar particles in the lungs break down the cilia, and this in turn impairs the ability of the bronchial tubes to propel mucus up towards the trachea and larynx so that coughing can get rid of it. It is because infections thrive in accumulated mucus that smokers have more bronchitis, influenza, sinusitis and emphysema than do non-smokers.

Carcinogens Research has yet to establish exactly which substances in cigarette smoke are cancer-causing, although top of the suspect list are eight which have been shown to cause cancer in animals.

Who still smokes?

Happily, smoking is on the decline among adults, although there is a worrying stability in the figures for the 11-to-15-year-old age group that bodes ill for the future. According to figures released by the Office of Population, Censuses and Surveys in September 1993, one child in 10 between the ages of 11 and 15 smokes, and that figure has not improved since 1990.

There are reckoned to be about 13.5 million adult smokers in Britain today and about 11 million ex-smokers. Over the decade 1980 to 1990, the proportion of smokers in the adult male population dropped from 42 per cent to 31 per cent and in females from 37 per cent to 29 per cent. Not only do more men than women still smoke, but in addition each man, on average, smokes more than the average woman. Around a quarter of the men who smoke and nearly a third of the women have tried at least once to quit.

Smoking and weight worries

Many smokers, particularly women, say they are reluctant to give up smoking because they are afraid they will gain weight, undesirable on both cosmetic and health grounds. The health argument doesn't hold water. You would have to gain about 10 stones (64kg) to put your health at the same degree of risk from obesity that you get from smoking 20 cigarettes a day. In fact, the average weight gain for smokers who give up the habit is about 4lb (2kg), and it is usually only temporary. You do hear horror stories about people putting on a stone or two, but if you cross-examine them about the extent to which they substituted sweets for cigarettes, it quickly becomes apparent that it was taking up sweets, not giving up cigarettes, that was to blame.

Smoking may help people keep their weight down a little. It can interfere with the digestive system so that smokers don't absorb energy from food properly. Smoking can suppress appetite, and it can dull your taste buds so food is less appealing. It also raises metabolic rate. Nevertheless, it doesn't follow that smoking makes you slim. One American study found that the fattest women on average were also the heaviest smokers.

When you stop smoking, getting plenty of extra exercise and being careful not to eat sweets as cigarette substitutes will help ensure that you do not fall into the weight-gain trap. If you find you crave something to put in your mouth when you are getting used to being an ex-smoker, go for something like celery or carrot sticks or a piece of fruit. You may find it helpful to have some crunchy vegetable nibbles prepared, ready for instant munching if the craving becomes urgent.

In fact, if you decide to blitz your health and make some of the simple changes to your life style and diet suggested in Chapters 1, 2 and 3 at the same time, you could end up not only a healthy non-smoker, but a slimmer and fitter one too.

Smoking and stress

Another reason many smokers say they are reluctant to give up is that a cigarette helps them relax. As noted above, this simply is not true. What really is happening is that, under stress, the body breaks down nicotine more quickly, which leads it to crave more. The relief from stress smokers think they experience with a cigarette is actually temporary relief from a craving set up by smoking itself. They will never be truly relaxed until they free themselves of that nicotine craving permanently.

Some smokers have got into the habit of stopping what they are doing from time to time to have a cigarette and to take a few minutes out for themselves. As they inhale, they begin to step back from their immediate problems to sort them through and put them in some sort of order of priority. Everything about that routine – except inhaling a lungful of noxious substances – is good stress management: stopping, taking a deep breath, exhaling slowly and fully are all sound steps in relieving stress (see Chapter 7 for fuller details).

A cigarette thus may seem relaxing to some smokers because inhaling smoke is the only time they really take a deep breath – taking in air (and, for them, smoke) right down into their lungs and then exhaling to the point of fully emptying their lungs. Deep breathing without the smoke, they can discover, is more relaxing still. It is therefore important that people giving up smoking think about other, smoke-free interludes of relaxation and deep breathing that they can build into their day. Not doing so can be the first step on the road to a relapse.

Pipes and cigars

Some cigarette smokers wonder if, instead of giving up smoking altogether, they can lengthen the odds in their favour by switching to a pipe or cigars. Coronary heart disease and lung cancer do pose less of a risk to pipe and cigar smokers than they do to cigarette smokers, although pipe and cigar smokers still are more at risk from these diseases than are non-smokers. It may be that what makes the difference is that cigarette smokers usually inhale, while cigar and pipe smokers usually only puff. However, cigar and pipe smokers are just as likely as cigarette smokers to get other cancers, such as cancer of the lip.

The bad news for cigarette smokers is that – although there is no actual proof of this – it is very unlikely that switching to a pipe or cigars would also cause them to shed the habit of inhaling. And continuing to inhale means they would probably fare no better than if they had continued to smoke cigarettes.

More reasons for giving up

The reasons outlined above are not the only ones for giving up the habit. If you are a smoker, stopping means:

- living longer
- sleeping better
- getting rid of smokers' cough
- improving stamina
- having a better sense of taste and of smell
- no longer having cigarette burns on clothes and furniture and reducing the risk of house fires
- saying goodbye to dirty, smelly ash trays
- finding paintwork, curtains and wallpaper staying cleaner and fresher for longer
- no longer having hair, clothes and skin that smell of stale tobacco smoke
- ending yellow stains on teeth and fingers
- saving money
- being able to wear contact lenses longer.

How to give up

According to a National Opinion Poll survey, the majority of adult smokers want to give up, and one in three of them are very keen to do so. Unfortunately, the survey also found that the more heavily people smoke the more they are convinced they cannot give up the habit.

Giving up is rarely easy. But large numbers of people do it every year. Not everyone is successful at the first attempt, but once you decide to do it, you can. Every time you try to give up and fail, you learn something that is valuable experience to draw on for the next attempt. If the first method does not work for you, the trick is to try another. Different methods work for different people.

The most important thing to remember is that, to stop and to stay stopped, you must realise that having just one cigarette is not a possibility – especially if you have been a regular (even if not particularly heavy) smoker. There are a few people who have a cigarette once in a while and then go days, weeks or even months without giving smoking another thought. They are rare, and they don't usually worry about giving up smoking because not smoking has never been an issue for them. But anyone who has been a regular daily smoker is extremely unlikely to be able to turn into that type of casual take-it-or-leave-it smoker the second time around.

A generally unsuccessful strategy is to try to give up by cutting down until you are smoking nothing at all. Some people do succeed that way. Most who try it don't. It is better, generally, to name the day you will throw the lot away – though there is no harm in getting your total down in preparation for that.

Most people find it helps to tell family, friends and colleagues at work that they plan to give up completely and when. That way, there is a certain pressure on them to live up to it. Here are some more tips that may help:

- Remember you are dealing with a triple agenda here. You are breaking an addiction to nicotine as well as the habit of lighting up. In addition, you have a new identity to get used to. You might be surprised to discover how much being a smoker is part of the way you see yourself.
- Keep a chart for a week beforehand of when you smoke, and rate each cigarette on a scale of 1 to 3, with 1 meaning you could have given it a miss without really suffering, 2 that it would have been pretty difficult to go without, and 3 as the one you'd have gone out and spent all night looking for rather than go without. Also mark for each cigarette what else was going on at the time – for example, making a telephone call, having coffee at the end of a meal, during or after a row, and so on. When you are preparing to give up, see what you can do either to avoid the situations in which you find yourself craving a cigarette rated 3, or to give yourself some sort of diversion or substitute treat, especially in the first couple of weeks.
- Remember that not everyone has withdrawal symptoms. Between 40 per cent and 50 per cent of those who give up don't. You just might find it easier than you expect.
- People who do have withdrawal symptoms – craving a cigarette, feeling irritable and finding it hard to concentrate are the most common – usually unintentionally make them worse by

hyperventilating. Deliberately slow down your breathing and breathe as deeply as you can, then empty your lungs completely again, to relieve them.

- Remember if you do find the going tough, your symptoms will not last more than a week or two, and the worst will be over in about three days. Then you can get on with the rest of your life – a smoke-free person.

- Remind yourself that the craving lasts only a few minutes at a time anyway. Instead of allowing it to be a signal to light up, use it as a nudge to do something different – drink a glass of water, telephone a friend, go for a walk, etc.

- Step up your exercise (or start some if you do not do any) in preparation. Studies have found that people who exercise have a better success rate when they attempt to give up smoking. It can help in a number of ways. It is better psychologically to do something active than to sit in front of the television set wallowing in thoughts of how much you want a cigarette. Brisk exercise will help you feel better physically more quickly. And it will help counteract any tendency to put on weight in the first weeks off the weed.

- Write down all your personal positive reasons for giving up and put them in order of importance to you. If you feel tempted to relapse, read the list through. Read it daily for the first couple of weeks anyway.

- Decide what, for you, would be the worst possible conse-quences of carrying on smoking. Dying, painfully of lung cancer? Not being around to see your grandchildren growing up? Struggling to get your breath with emphysema? Having a leg amputated? Again, you might like to write down all the consequences you fear and rank them in order. Use this list the same way as the one above.

- Watch your alcohol intake for the first couple of weeks. Better still, cut it out. Not only do many people have a pattern of smoking when they drink, but alcohol also saps willpower.

- If you always have a cigarette with coffee, it may help to switch to drinking tea or a cold drink and giving the coffee a miss for a week or two as well.

- Drink eight to ten glasses of water a day to begin with. It helps flush the nicotine out of your system and halves the time it takes for those people who do crave cigarettes to get over it. Drinking water leaves a clean taste in your mouth, too.

- If you know you are going to miss having something to put in your mouth, make sure you have an instant supply of low-fat, healthy substitutes to chew, such as scraped and chopped-up carrot sticks and slices of celery. Reaching for sweets or biscuits will only pile on the weight.
- Decide what you are going to do with the money you save by giving up smoking. You might decide to put the cost of your day's smoking into a jar each day, towards a luxury holiday or new clothes.
- Find a friend who wants to give up, too, and offer one another support. Promise each other that if either feels tempted, he or she will phone the other.
- If you feel like having a cigarette, brush your teeth instead.
- Avoid the company of smokers as much as you can, especially for the first couple of weeks.
- Spend as much time at first as you reasonably can in places where you cannot smoke.
- Vary your routine as much as possible for the first week or so.
- If you weaken and have one cigarette, it doesn't mean you should give up the attempt, or even postpone it until the next day. Many people successfully give up even after one or two lapses.
- Remember every day that it will be a little easier the next day.
- Take it a day at a time.

Help to quit
Besides your own willpower, there are a number of sources of extra help that you might want to consider trying. Hard data on relative effectiveness is hard to come by for most, but there is anecdotal evidence that each kind of help works for some people. Be wary, however, of anyone offering a 90 per cent success rate: that is highly unlikely to be true. Choices include the following:

Acupuncture Acupuncturists either insert needles into the ear and leave them in situ for the patient to twiddle when they feel the urge to smoke, or remove needles at the end of each session of a course of treatment. They might suggest you come back for a booster session if something particularly stressful crops up in your life in the first few months. Find a qualified practitioner through the Council for Acupuncture★, the British Acupuncture Association★ or the Traditional Acupuncture Society★. Some doctors also offer acupuncture at their surgeries.

Dummy cigarettes Sold in many shops including pharmacies, dummy cigarettes look like the real thing but are plastic and you don't light them. The idea is that they give some taste satisfaction when drawn like a cigarette, but they don't provide any nicotine. There is no evidence for or against their effectiveness. They have no known side effects.

Groups There are various groups for people attempting to give up smoking, and these can offer information, advice and mutual support to members. Approaches vary, but there are usually something between five and eight sessions of one to two hours, led by someone with some training in counselling and motivation, or by a doctor or practice nurse. Leaders are often, though not always, ex-smokers themselves. Costs vary from nothing or a token charge to quite high commercial rates. If you cannot find a group through your local library, your doctor or Quitline★, you could always form your own.

Herbal cigarettes You can replace ordinary cigarettes with herbal ones. The idea is then to cut down on them too. They contain no nicotine and less carbon monoxide and tar than ordinary cigarettes do. There is no evidence, however, that if people do use them long term they would be safe.

Hypnosis Hypnotherapists use the pleasantly relaxed state of trance to support people in their intention to give up smoking by giving suggestions to their subconscious minds. Some also teach self-hypnosis, which gives ex-smokers an alternative way to deal with stress and teaches them to relax.

Usually only a few sessions are needed, although if smoking proves persistent, a hypnotherapist might then explore what role smoking is fulfilling for a smoker which needs to be met in another way. Some doctors offer hypnosis. Or it is possible to find a qualified hypnotherapist through the National Council of Psychotherapists and Hypnotherapy Register★ or the Institute for Complementary Medicine★.

Nicotine products Gum (available over the counter from pharmacies or on prescription) can help curb withdrawal symptoms and possibly cigarette cravings if it is used properly. Research has found skin patches (available over the counter from pharmacies) help in the short term, though long-term trials are needed on them. There is no evidence either way yet on lozenges and tablets (sold widely, including by pharmacies). Side effects, however, have been reported with all three types of product, ranging from mild jaw ache from chewing the gum to disturbed sleep, vivid dreams and skin rashes from patches. There is also some danger of addiction.

Non-nicotine products These include capsules that have been shown to have short-term success, although no information is available about longer-term results. Silver acetate products make a cigarette taste so revolting that you will want to put it out. Filters take out some of the tar and nicotine from smoke, and some claim to help you cut down. Then there are other products that contain tobacco flavouring and vitamins, and herbal anti-smoking tablets which contain lobelia, supposed to have a tobacco-like effect. There are no known side effects and no evidence that these products are harmful to take; nor is there any evidence, so far, that they work.

Alcohol

Year by year, the case against having any tobacco at all grows. But drinking a little of your favourite tipple has been given a rather cleaner bill of health for most of us by recent research.

Moderate drinkers seem to fare better than those who drink nothing, according to a number of studies. Among them have been two large-scale 10-year studies which found that people who drank up to two drinks a day were less likely to have a heart attack than those who did not drink at all. Another major report found that people who had only a couple of drinks a day had slightly lower blood pressure than teetotallers.

However, there is a possibility that these studies exaggerate the benefits a little. Non-drinkers include – as well as people who have never touched a drop in their lives – alcoholics in recovery, people who have been advised to give up because of some medical problem, and people who have chosen to stop because they felt alcohol did not agree with them in some way. Most studies do not make this distinction and so their results may be biased somewhat towards the benefits of moderate drinking.

Some epidemiologists believe wine may be the reason the French have lower coronary heart disease rates than the British do, despite a high consumption of animal fats, especially in such products as cheese. *The Lancet*, in January 1993, took the argument one stage further by suggesting that it was red wine rather than white that could protect the heart, and that the reason could be powerful anti-oxidants (explained in Chapter 3) called procyanidins found in it.

However, even if it is true that drinking more red wine does provide some protection against heart disease for the French, there is no net gain. They are more likely than the British to die from alcohol-related liver disease and in alcohol-related road accidents.

Recent research suggests that moderate drinking might be beneficial for the brain as well as the body. A 20-year study at the Indiana School of Medicine in the US has followed 4000 male twins who served in the US Army during the Second World War and who are now aged between 66 and 76. It found that people who took one or two drinks a day had less deterioration of reasoning, problem-solving and other cognitive skills with age than either non-drinkers or heavy drinkers.

At the moment, there does not seem any compelling health case for moderate drinkers to feel they ought to give up this pleasure, and there may well be some benefit in it. However, it is a different story for heavier drinkers, who, studies show, have a higher risk of coronary heart disease. Too much alcohol can also raise blood pressure and lead to weight problems and hence greater risk of all the obesity-related illnesses.

What is alcohol?

Alcohol acts as a drug. In small doses, it relaxes the body, increases appetite and produces, in most healthy people, a feeling of well-being. In larger doses, it becomes a powerful poison. Some estimates attribute 10 per cent of all deaths to it, either from the physical consequences of long-term over-indulgence or from the accidents it causes.

Alcohol has no essential nutrients at all, and actually has an adverse effect on nutrition because it can deplete the body's sources of some minerals and vitamins, or make them less readily absorbed. It is the enemy of the overweight because it is simply empty calories and tends to stimulate appetite as well.

When you have a drink, 95 per cent of the alcohol is absorbed directly into the bloodstream, and within minutes it has gone to every part of the body that contains water – lungs, kidneys, heart and brain. The effect on the brain is at first to remove inhibitions, but as more is absorbed it becomes sedative or depressant. Reaction time, co-ordination, eyesight and the ability to judge depth deteriorate quickly. Drinking too much will induce sleep.

In fact, alcohol slows down metabolism, breathing and circulation, and there comes a point where it will paralyse breathing completely, with fatal consequences – although it is rare for the body not to protect itself by vomiting or ensuring the drinker passes out and so has to stop drinking. Enzymes in the liver break down the alcohol in the bloodstream, but this takes time. There is no shortcut to sobering up. Black coffee and cold showers don't help at all.

When we experience a hangover, what we are feeling is the body's attempts to repair itself. Blood vessels in the brain, which had become dilated while the alcohol was around, give you a headache as they return to normal. Gastric juices altered by the presence of alcohol make themselves felt as stomach upsets. The overstimulated kidneys excrete too much water, resulting in dehydration. The only treatments for a hangover are sleep, aspirin, plenty of liquids, eating something bland, and time. For every unit of alcohol drunk, the body needs about two hours to detoxify – which explains why a driver can still be over the legal limit the morning after.

What is moderate?
It is impossible to say exactly what constitutes a safe level of drinking for any individual. Some people drink far more than the recommended guidelines all their lives and seem to suffer no ill effects. Some drink less, yet still become so dependent on alcohol that they face a stark choice between giving up drink completely and giving up on their hopes of a normal, healthy life. In general

terms, however, the guidelines believed to be a safe upper limit for most people are as follows:

- **Men** should have no more than 21 units a week, spread over five or six days, with one or two alcohol-free days (see chart below for definition of 'a unit').
- **Women** should have no more than 14 units a week, similarly spread over five or six days, with one or two days without alcohol each week.

Remember these figures are not a 'recommended daily dose'. They are a recommended upper limit.

If you need to cut down, it might help if you try the following:

- Alternate alcoholic drinks with non-alcoholic.
- Dilute drinks with mixers, mineral water or tap water.
- Try to drink more slowly – consciously make yourself take smaller sips, spaced further apart.
- Don't drink alcohol when you are thirsty; have a glass of water, fruit juice or soft drink first.
- Don't drink on an empty stomach.
- Avoid salty nibbles such as crisps and nuts.
- Deliberately decide on and stick to drink-free days once or twice a week.
- Don't become discouraged if you cut down and find you are becoming constipated (increasing the fibre and non-alcoholic liquids in your diet will sort that out).

KNOW YOUR DRINKS

Alcohol intake is measured in units. One unit =

| ½ pint of ordinary lager, beer or cider | ¼ pint of strong lager, beer or cider | 1 small glass of sherry or fortified wine | 1 single pub measure of spirits | 1 small glass of table wine |

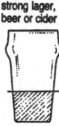 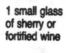

ALCOHOL: HOW MUCH PER WEEK?

Units	Men	Women
below 14	////	////
15–21	////	::::
22–35	::::	■■■■
36+	■■■■	■■■■

//// = acceptable but have one or two alcohol-free days in the week

:::: = in the danger zone: try to drink less

■■■■ = dangerous: cut down immediately – your drinking could do long-term damage to your health

If you know you are drinking more than you should and more than you want, and you find you just cannot cut back, Alcohol Concern★ can give details of treatment and advice centres near you, and Alcoholics Anonymous★ (AA) is the largest and best-known of the self-help groups. Al-Anon★ offers support to the partners and friends of alcoholics, and Alateen★ does so to their children.

Coffee and tea

Caffeine, like alcohol, is a drug – one of the family called xanthines which occur naturally in about 60 species of plant. It can be found in coffee beans, tea leaves, cocoa seeds and the cola nut. No one knows why plants make it, but one theory is that it is a natural herbicide which gives them an evolutionary edge over the competition for the same environmental niche.

The effect of caffeine on the human body is complex and fast-acting. It is easily absorbed in the gut and in minutes has travelled via the blood to all the tissues and organs of the body.

Caffeine molecules fit themselves on to brain receptors designed to take another chemical called adenosine, which is a natural sedative that tells the cells of the body to slow down. By interfering with adenosine functioning, caffeine shifts the body into top gear. Blood pressure, central nervous system activity and urine output all increase. Breathing becomes faster, muscles become stronger and the blood vessels in the brain constrict. Not for nothing has caffeine been called the most widely used behaviour-modifying drug in the world.

Many of us tend to think of coffee and caffeine as almost synonymous, but there is more caffeine per ounce in tea. It is only because less tea than coffee goes into the average cup that a cup of coffee tends to contain more. The stronger the tea brews, the more caffeine it contains. The variety of tea plant and the production method used will also affect its caffeine content. Different types of coffee also have different caffeine levels, and a strong cup of tea can have more caffeine than a weak cup of coffee. There is also caffeine in some soft drinks, in chocolate and in some medicines.

If the instant charge we get from a cup of coffee makes us feel that our thought processes have improved, we may be kidding ourselves. Studies so far have been unable to show any evidence of improved intellectual or learning performance.

Nor does a cup of black coffee help us to sober up. It anything, it makes us worse because it is a diuretic and so increases dehydration. If it is hot coffee, it is worse still, since hot drinks increase the rate at which the bloodstream absorbs alcohol. Far from sobering up someone who has drunk too much, hot black coffee will make him or her more drunk.

The case against coffee

Serious charges have been laid against coffee. But the worst verdict the present evidence could support against most coffee is not entirely proven. More than 20 published studies have found a link between coffee drinking and raised levels of blood cholesterol, with a consequent increased risk of coronary heart disease. One study, published in Norway and reported in the *British Medical Journal* in March 1990, came to the even gloomier conclusion that there was an increased risk of heart disease beyond the effect that could be attributed to the increased level of cholesterol.

However, studies have contradicted one another. Some have been flawed by a failure to separate out the effects of smoking and coffee drinking. Often, researchers have not looked at whether coffee drinkers were taking milk or cream and so increasing their intake of fat compared with volunteers who did not drink coffee, and studies have also failed to tease out such subtle factors as personality and life style.

The most reliable finding seems to be that a link between increased blood cholesterol and consequently a higher risk of coronary heart disease is confined to coffee made of boiled grounds and drunk strong, black and unfiltered the way it is in the Scandinavian countries but not usually in Britain. Instant and filtered coffee and tea do not seem to have the same adverse effect. Attempts to find a link between coffee and diabetes and various cancers have been inconclusive.

However, there are other reasons you might want to consider cutting coffee out of your diet, or cutting down on it. Too much can interfere with a good night's sleep and can cause frayed tempers, nervousness, palpitations, stomach upsets, nausea, tinnitus and pre-menstrual syndrome. Our tolerance of caffeine declines with age, although regular coffee drinkers seem to become somewhat desensitised to the effects.

If you find you are feeling irrationally anxious or having panic attacks, you might be advised to try cutting coffee right out of your diet for a time to see what difference it makes. If you do, don't be disappointed if the first change you notice is a headache. Persist until it goes. Even a slight decrease in regular intake can be enough to trigger one. The withdrawal symptoms usually last only a few days, after which most people report feeling better than they did when they were drinking coffee.

Doctors generally recommend a maximum intake – even for people who do not feel they are suffering any ill effects – of about 400mg a day, which is about four mugs or six cups of coffee. People with raised blood pressure, kidney disease, high cholesterol or a history of heart disease should have less. Decaffeinated coffee is a large and growing market, despite the fact that tea and coffee also contain a number of other active chemical substances besides caffeine, any or all of which could be guilty of the adverse effects coffee has been found to have on some people.

Caffeine can be removed in one of several ways. Organic solvents such as methylene chloride or ethyl acetate can be used to dissolve the caffeine out of green coffee beans. Another method is to put moistened beans in a chamber with liquid carbon dioxide, which has the ability to remove caffeine without affecting other natural chemicals in coffee or tea.

Then there is the Swiss Water Process, in which hot water is used to wash out caffeine. A variant on that is the European Water Process, in which the caffeine-rich solution in the Swiss Water Process is treated with organic solvent. (Water processes aren't suitable for tea.)

Manufacturers don't have to say on the label which method they have used, although those who don't use organic solvents tend to choose to draw attention to the fact.

Smoking and drinking: a summary

The best available advice on stimulants is simple:

- Smoking is a real killer.
- A little alcohol probably does more good than harm for most of us.
- A moderate intake of coffee (as long as it has not been boiled) probably does no real harm. But you might find your physical and mental health improve if you cut it down or out.

CHAPTER 5

TIME OF CHANGE

UNDERSTANDING the inevitable physical changes that take place as we grow older enables us to cope better with them. It helps us to accept these changes for what they are – part of a normal healthy life cycle – and to make informed decisions about the most appropriate way for us to manage them. This is true whether we are confronting problems in our sexual relationships, choices about late parenthood, the symptoms of the menopause or worries about the loss of youthful potency.

For women, the menopause marks a watershed in their lives. It is nature's confirmation that they can no longer bear children, at least not without the help of controversial new technology. That can make it a landmark of profound psychological significance. For some women, it brings a real sense of liberation, while others find it deeply depressing, and some start by feeling negative only to discover gradually the plus side. Most have a response that falls somewhere in-between.

For men, the physiological equivalent of the female menopause comes more slowly. There is no sudden cut-off point to pull them up sharply with the realisation of transition into a new phase. But falling hormone levels, or perhaps a failing efficiency at putting hormones to work, may have their psychological impact on their lives, too.

Sex after 40

A good sex life is one that satisfies both partners – whether that means intercourse unfailingly several times a week or putting the emphasis more on kisses, cuddles and skin contact. It is not about living up to the expectations or matching the real or imagined performance of others. It is about pleasing yourself and one another.

For some couples, the middle years of their lives bring a real sexual liberation. Being in a trusting and settled relationship, freedom from fear of unplanned pregnancy, nights no longer broken by the needs and demands of small children – it can all add up to a new phase of less-troubled sexuality.

Unfortunately, this isn't necessarily so.

The sexual problems men can encounter in their middle years include loss of libido and difficulties in physical performance such as getting and keeping an erection (erectile impotence). Erectile impotence can be a side effect of some illnesses such as diabetes; it can be caused by drinking too much, or tranquillisers; or it can result from medication (prescribed, for example, for high blood pressure or sleep problems).

If it is not a side effect of an illness or medication, erectile impotence can be either psychological or physical in cause, and the first step towards treating it is to determine which. In fact, it is rarely quite as clear-cut as that suggests. A physical cause may be identified in about 50 per cent of impotent men, but it is often complicated by an additional emotional component, and treatment may need to focus on both aspects.

Although the effect of the hormone testosterone on sex drive is still disputed (see the section on the male menopause, below), it is generally thought that whatever effect it does have must be through its action on the sexual centres of the brain, rather than directly on the body. When testosterone levels are very low, a supplement may be prescribed.

Otherwise, the next stage of investigation will be to determine whether the physical problem lies in the functioning of the nerves in the penis which dilate the arteries and increase the blood flowing into the columns of tissue running along the penis to increase its volume – or in the blood-flow itself. Treatment is usually by injection of drugs directly into the penis, or by a penile implant with either a hinging or inflating mechanism by which an erection can be switched on and off again. *The Which? Guide to Men's Health**, published by Consumers' Association, gives more details on methods of treating impotence problems.

The Kegel pelvic floor exercises (see box on p.124) prove helpful for some men with impotence difficulties. Sometimes the most helpful therapy for those experiencing sexual difficulties can be the realisation that sex in the middle years can improve in proportion to the time made available. Erection and arousal may just take longer than they did before.

Women around and after the time of the menopause may also experience difficulties, including feeling less sexually responsive, discomfort during intercourse, lower libido and loss of interest in their sexual partners. For them, oestrogen replacement can help with a range of physiological factors, from the maintenance of a healthy vagina to sensitivity to touch. So can a gentle, patient and considerate partner.

An active sex life can also play a major role in keeping a woman's sexual organs in good working condition. Use of a lubricant or a moisturiser can also ease intercourse. (Petroleum jelly is not recommended because it is not water soluble and could get into the vagina or urethra and cause irritation.)

As with the emotional difficulties women can experience around the time of the menopause (see section on the female menopause, below), their sexual problems may be complicated by a number of factors. Interest in sex may be reduced not as a direct result of the menopause, but in the wake of other symptoms, including tiredness, irritability and depression, or as a side effect of medication, or in some cases as a response to her partner's apparent loss of interest.

Long-standing sexual disappointments and dissatisfactions on either side may boil over when his or her menopausal symptoms become the last straw for stressed relationships. A contributing factor to sexual difficulties for a woman going through the menopause may be resentment of or unhappiness about her male partner's erection or other problems. He may then exacerbate her unhappiness by abstaining from physical contact. Equally, a man going through a mid-life crisis of his own may take it as a slur on his sexual attractiveness if his wife is suffering a loss of libido. He may turn elsewhere for reassurance, putting the relationship in even greater jeopardy.

The picture, overall, may not be as gloomy as that sounds. When John McKinlay, Professor of Sociology and Epidemiology at Boston University, analysed the experiences of a random group of 1700 men aged between 40 and 70, he found that their expectations of sex declined with age, but not their levels of satisfaction.

However, if average sexual satisfaction does not necessarily decline, many couples could have happier relationships if they become willing to talk more openly to one another about their desires. They can also seek help from their doctors, or from an organisation such as Relate*, when things do go wrong for them physically or emotionally, or in their relationship.

If you are reluctant to seek outside help for your difficulties, you may find it helpful to remember that you are extremely unlikely to be able to tell any doctor or therapist anything he or she has not heard before. (See Chapter 7 for advice on how to find a therapist.)

Difficulties in coping with stress also have a particularly insidious habit of spilling over into other areas of our lives, especially into our bedrooms, making sleep difficult or disturbed and interfering with the pleasures of sex. Chapter 7, which considers how to evaluate and manage the sources of stress in our lives, could have a useful spin-off for your sex life.

Pregnancy after 40

If most women have most of their children before they reach the age of 40, not all do. Recent research suggests that about one in 20 of these 'late' mothers are so by choice – they have made a deliberate decision to postpone having children until this last-chance time.

For the majority of them, there are other reasons why motherhood comes later rather than sooner. They may have been unable to have a baby earlier because of fertility problems, or may not have been in a stable relationship. And some later pregnancies take their owners by surprise. Family doctors are familiar with the consultation that begins with a woman telling them she thinks she must be approaching the menopause, and ends with a positive pregnancy test.

Although fertility begins to fall at about age 25, with the decline becoming significant by around 35, there are women who appear to have a sudden and unexplained increase in fertility, sometimes described as 'the last fling of the ovaries', around the age of 39.

This is claimed to explain at least some of the grandmothers and mothers of teenaged families who are surprised to find themselves pregnant again at around the age of 40.

There are slightly higher risks, on average, for older mothers. But to put them in perspective, the increase is small and the risks are also higher for those aged under 20. Part of the greater risk, moreover, simply reflects the statistical fact that older women are more likely to have a number of conditions, including diabetes and cardiovascular disease, which make pregnancy riskier at any age. The risk statistics have to be read in the light of all these things.

Nevertheless, there is a greater statistical danger for older women of having a baby with Down's syndrome. The risk increases, on average, as shown in Table 1.

However, chromosomal abnormalities such as Down's syndrome and such conditions as spina bifida can be detected by amniocentesis. This test analyses a sample of amniotic fluid from the uterus and is offered routinely to pregnant women aged around 35 or so (depending on local hospital policy) and over. The test is done between weeks 16 and 22, and there is then a four-week wait for the results.

Amniocentesis does involve a slightly increased risk of miscarriage, while a non–invasive blood test (called the maternal screening or 'triple test') does not. Nor, however, is the blood test as revealing: it identifies only who is at higher-than-average risk of having a baby with Down's syndrome. Some mothers-to-be

Table 1: INCIDENCE OF DOWN'S SYNDROME BY AGE OF MOTHER

Age	Incidence
25	1 in 1500
30	1 in 800
35	1 in 350
36	1 in 300
37	1 in 200
38	1 in 170
39	1 in 140
40	1 in 100
45	1 in 30

decide to have a triple test first, and to opt for amniocentesis only if the first test indicates high risk for them.

Older mothers are also slightly more at risk – but again only on average – of miscarriage or of having a premature baby. And studies have found an apparently higher incidence of complications of pregnancy and labour in older than in younger mothers, although there is also evidence that at least some of this increase may simply reflect the medical profession's tendency to intervene more readily by inducing delivery or delivering by Caesarian section when they are dealing with older mothers.

Physically, a fit woman in her 20s is probably hitting the peak time for pregnancy. Her body is mature and strong, yet still supple. But psychologically and socially, the older mother may have the edge. She may be more settled in herself, more established in her career and under less financial pressure than she would have been a decade or two earlier. In addition, a fit 40-year-old in good health who takes sensible care of herself and her diet is actually likely to fare better through pregnancy than one in her 20s or early 30s who is less fit and careful.

There is more detailed information about pregnancy at 40 and beyond in *The National Childbirth Trust Book of Pregnancy, Birth and Parenthood*★★ edited by Glynnis Tucker and *Better Late than Never*★★ written by Maggie Jones. The National Childbirth Trust★ also has a number of leaflets about pregnancy.

The female menopause

The word 'menopause' is derived from two Greek roots: *men* meaning month, and *pausis*, meaning cessation, and it refers to the ends of menstruation and of fertility – two events in a woman's life which may not happen at exactly the same time. The whole process may last from one year to seven. Most women stop having periods between ages 49 and 51, although it can be as early as the mid-30s or as late as the mid-60s. The menopause is just one phase of the climacteric, another word of Greek origin (literally 'rung of the ladder'). The climacteric describes the time before, during and after the menopause when ovary function and the production of hormones decline and the body re-adapts.

Menstrual cycle

To understand the female menopause, it is necessary to understand something of the chemical changes involved in the cycle that recurs monthly throughout a woman's fertile years. Because the cycle is a recurring one, it has no real beginning or end. But it can be thought of as starting with a message from the hypothalamus, an endocrine gland which sends its chemical message to the pituitary gland, another endocrine gland just below it in the brain.

In response, the pituitary secretes follicle-stimulating hormone, or FSH, and some luteinising hormone, or LH, and sends these messengers on their way to the ovaries. During the first half of the cycle, it is the FSH that ripens an egg in an ovarian follicle before it finds its way into the fallopian tube at ovulation, about halfway through the cycle.

The developing ovarian follicles are lined with cells which produce both a protein-like substance called inhibin and the hormone oestrogen, and release them into the bloodstream. The rising oestrogen level has a powerful effect on the lining of the uterus (the endometrium), which thickens and becomes rich in blood vessels. The rising level of inhibin reduces the amount of FSH being produced by the pituitary. This in turn puts LH production into a higher gear. The ripe egg is actually released in response to a surge of LH.

After the egg is released, the left-over follicle produces a large quantity of progesterone and a small amount of oestrogen. Progesterone makes the new tissue that has been laid down in the endometrium in response to the oestrogen softer and more sponge-like, ready to receive a fertilised egg.

If the egg is not fertilised by a rendezvous with live male sperm, then three or four days before the start of the period, production of both hormones declines and the uterus sheds the lining that had been prepared to provide a suitable environment for an embryo. When the hypothalamus signals to the pituitary gland that the hormones are at their lowest, the pituitary sends FSH to the ovaries and the whole cycle starts up again.

Women start life with about two million immature egg cells in their ovaries and still have around 300,000 potential eggs at puberty. The rest have already been lost by natural wastage. By the

HORMONE CHANGES DURING THE MENSTRUAL CYCLE

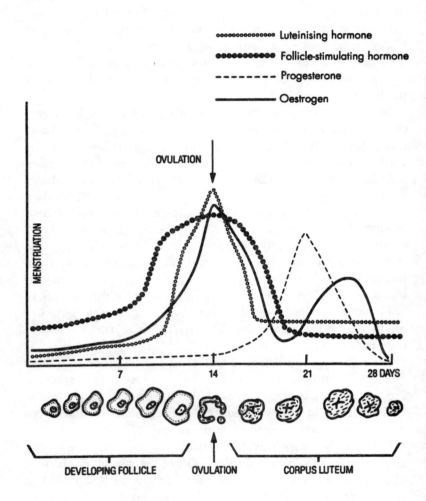

time we are 40, we have only about 50 left. As the numbers decline, some months may pass without ovulation or menstruation, or the production of post-ovulation oestrogen or progesterone, before the eventual menopause, when all the eggs have been used up.

During this period of the peri-menopause, menstrual flow may alter to become lighter or heavier, and the cycle is likely to be irregular. Once the lining of the uterus is no longer being shed regularly, when it does disintegrate and come away it can do so in uneven patches, causing heavier or more erratic periods for a time. (Although irregular periods are to be expected, irregular bleeding is not. Bleeding between periods, after intercourse or more than six months after the menopause should be reported to and investigated by your doctor.)

Oestrogen production remains near-normal in the early years of the peri-menopause, so symptoms such as hot flushes and vaginal dryness are not yet felt. As oestrogen and progesterone levels fall, the pituitary gland desperately tries to kick-start production again by releasing ever increasing levels of FSH and LH into the blood. In fact, FSH can get up to 13 times and LH to three times normal levels. These elevated levels provide doctors with a means of testing for the approach of the menopause. Testing is not done routinely. Age and symptoms are enough to indicate when most women are at or near the menopause. But it can be useful, for example, to check the suspected early onset of menopause.

When the ovaries stop producing eggs, they stop making progesterone and secrete only much smaller amounts of oestrogen, but the adrenal glands and some other sources, including fat cells in the skin, continue to make a little contribution to the oestrogen levels too. Eventually, the follicles no longer respond at all to the FSH and LH. Oestrogen and progesterone levels fall too low for the uterine lining to grow at all, and the menopause occurs.

However, the ovaries still produce hormones that are converted into oestrone, a form of oestrogen, and some women still have oestrone in their blood 20 years after the menopause. For most, the adrenal glands become the major source of oestrogen after the menopause. Body fat is also involved in converting another hormone, androstenedione, into oestrone in muscle, the liver,

THE FEMALE REPRODUCTIVE SYSTEM

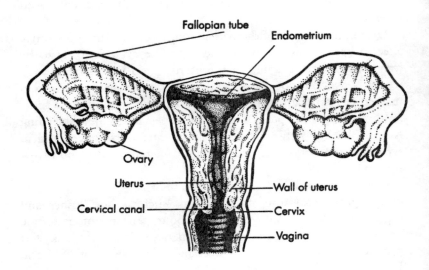

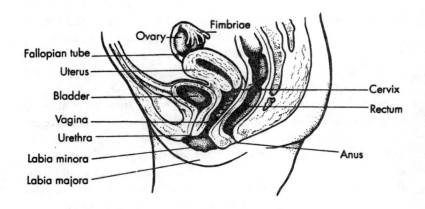

kidneys, brain and possibly at other (still undiscovered) sites. Interestingly, plumper women have a later menopause on average than thinner women, and report less discomfort when they do.

Although oestrogen has a profound effect on the body, including acting directly on the nervous system, it is probably not responsible for all the changes that occur around the time of the menopause. Hot flushes, night sweats, vaginal dryness, thinning of the tissues, loss of elasticity in the skin and of calcium in bone are related to hormone levels. But at least some sag and spread are probably more a product of lack of fitness and the passage of time than the passing of oestrogen. Many of the more psychological symptoms such as impatience, anxiety and feeling down in the dumps may be physical, mental or an interaction between the two.

Symptoms of the menopause

About one woman in five sails through the menopause with little or nothing in the way of symptoms of the changes taking place in her body. For the rest, the severity of symptoms varies.

Physical symptoms encountered around the time of the menopause include the following:

Altered menstrual flow See p.121.

Vaginal dryness This symptom can cause painful intercourse, and a risk of bleeding and infection. There is also shrinkage of the uterus (or womb) and the cervix (neck of the womb), and shortening of the cervical canal.

Shrinkage of the bladder and urethra The urethra is the passage that leads out of the body from the bladder. Its shrinkage, along with atrophy of the trigone of the bladder (the doorkeeper to the urethra), can cause a pressing need to pass urine frequently and sometimes to incontinence after sneezing or coughing. The involuntary loss of urine with the sudden urge to urinate responds well to Kegel exercises (see box on p.124) to improve the surrounding muscles. Involuntary loss with coughing, sneezing or laughing may need surgical or other muscle-strengthening correction.

Kegel exercises

In order to get the feel of where your sphincter muscle is, all you do is to stop the flow of urine while you are urinating. That contracts it. Before you start doing the exercises below, practise stopping and starting a few times at will so you become familiar with the feel of that muscle contracting and relaxing.

Then, contract the muscle for three seconds and release it for one. Contract and release five more times, making each contraction three seconds long and each release one second long. Repeat the lot three times a day for a few days. Then repeat the pattern 12 times a day for a week.

Skin and hair changes You might notice your skin becoming drier and thinner, your nails more brittle and hair thinner and drier from the peri-menopause onwards. In the first 10 years after the menopause, women lose 30 per cent of the collagen which forms a large part of the skin's connective support tissue. This leaves the skin even thinner, more easily bruised and with a more transparent, waxy look to it. Oestrogen replacement (see under hormone replacement therapy, below) restores lost collagen to pre-menopausal levels within six months. It increases the water content of the skin and improves the blood supply to it, and promotes the growth of thicker, healthier-looking hair. Some menopausal women suffer from a dry throat, burning mouth and problems with swallowing caused by lack of water content in and blood supply to tissues in the mouth and throat. Again, oestrogen replacement can help with this.

Hot flushes, night sweats and palpitations Probably the most familiar symptoms of the menopause are what are called the vaso-motor symptoms, which are caused by the changing size of blood vessels triggered by fluctuations in oestrogen levels before the menopause. About 80 per cent of women experience just before and around the time of the menopause hot flushes, night sweats and palpitations, as well as the headaches that can result from lack of sleep because of flushes and sweats. No one understands exactly what causes them, but it is probably something to do with a breakdown in the temperature control by the hypothalamus as oestrogen production declines. Oestrogen replacement usually eases these vasomotor symptoms within 10 days, although some people find it is two or three months before they fully feel the benefits. (Non-hormonal approaches are also discussed below.)

Changes in the breasts Breasts may become smaller and the nipples smaller and flatter around the time of the menopause. The areola may darken a little and skin may become rougher and thinner.

Loss of bone mass Bone mass reduces more rapidly at and after the menopause, which may lead eventually to osteoporosis, a condition in which some older women (and, eventually, older men) become more susceptible to fractures. It can also cause loss of height and deformity of the spine. If you take any group of 70-year-old women, for example, you can expect a tenth of them to have a hip fracture over the following five years. Between one in ten and one in five of those who do break a hip will die as a result. Only between a quarter and a half of the women who survive such fractures regain the level of functioning they had before; and many women with osteoporosis have several fractures.

Vulnerability to bone loss seems to be increased by a number of factors, including premature menopause, osteoporosis in the family, heavy drinking, smoking, being small-boned, not having enough calcium in earlier years, lack of exercise, long-term use of some drugs (particularly steroids) and too much caffeine. Genetics also play a role. Women of African origin, for example, tend to have much stronger bones to start with and so lose bone less than, for example, Asian and Caucasian women do. Screening to check bone density is possible but expensive and not widely used. Hormone replacement therapy seems both to stop bone loss while it is being taken and to slow the rate of loss for some years after it is stopped (although exercise is still the best protection for bones).

Cardiovascular changes Blood vessels, too, change at and after the time of the menopause, and women become more at risk from heart disease. Degree of risk is determined by family history, and increases with high blood pressure, diabetes, smoking, obesity, lack of exercise, a competitive personality and an unhealthy diet –

125

i.e. one that is high in saturated fat and low in fruit, vegetables, starch and fibre.

Besides these physical symptoms, most women report a number of emotional changes around the time of the menopause. These include mood swings, irritability, anxiety, memory difficulties, loss of concentration, tiredness and depression. Studies have attempted, with rather limited success, to tease apart the role of physiological factors triggered mostly by the loss of oestrogen (including sleep disturbance caused by hot flushes and night sweats) from the role of psychological factors such as what a woman believes about menopause and how she is dealing with what else is going on in her life at the same time. Children may be growing up and becoming more independent, even leaving home, leaving her grieving for her lost maternal role. Encroaching wrinkles may worry a woman who sees them as a sign that her best years are over. She may be worried about finding or keeping a place in a competitive and often youth-biased job market.

A number of cross-cultural studies have also attempted to establish how differences in attitude to ageing and expectations about the menopause might be related to the symptoms women suffer, also with ambiguous results. Women in Indian villages in Peru, for example, actually look forward to the menopause, for it is a time when they are freed from reproductive duties and become more socially and politically powerful. In fact, when Yewoubdar Beyene, an anthropologist at the University of California, questioned women in their late 40s and early 50s about hot flushes, she was met with blank stares of incomprehension.

Yet studies of women on the Greek island of Evia, who also live in a culture with positive attitudes towards ageing and who have had similarly large families to those of the women studied in Peru, found the Greek women suffered the same menopausal symptoms as women in industrialised Western countries.

Japanese women, too, it used to be thought, may have had fewer problems with the menopause because it was traditionally considered a sign of becoming wise and respectable there. But the Japanese diet is rich in foods such as tofu and miso, both made from soya beans, which contain oestrogen. It now looks as if this dietary 'hormone replacement therapy' actually deserves at least some of the credit.

However much of a role expectations are eventually found to play (or not) in the experience of menopause, women in America, where hot flushes are called hot flashes, have taken the initiative on attitude. They have framed notices on their office walls saying, 'I don't have hot flashes. I have power surges.'

Hormone replacement therapy

Hormone replacement therapy (HRT) has been hailed across the Atlantic as the greatest thing since sliced bread. About 80 per cent of women with menopausal symptoms in the US and Canada have taken it. The UK has responded more cautiously. The figure is only about 10 per cent, though Britain has been in the forefront of menopausal research in general and safe HRT techniques in particular.

Some family doctors are still more likely to give women complaining of menopause symptoms a prescription for a tranquilliser or sedative than counselling about HRT, and will refer to a gynaecologist or special menopause clinic only those patients who lobby strongly for it. Other general practitioners are enthusiastic about HRT and offer it freely, even routinely.

HRT goes back to the 1950s, when it was just oestrogen, without progesterone, and was prescribed for hot flushes, sweats, vaginal dryness, joint discomfort and urinary problems. We now know the first women who took it had fewer strokes and heart attacks and less osteoporosis as well.

By the 1960s, it had become clear that, for those women who had not had a hysterectomy, oestrogen on its own was not the whole answer. Taking just oestrogen, without a synthetic progesterone called progestogen as well, increases the risk of hyperplasia, or thickening of the lining of the uterus, which can be a forerunner of endometrial cancer. Adding progestogen to the cycle for seven days a month reduces the increased hyperplasia risk from between 7 and 15 per cent to 5 per cent, and progestogen for 12 to 13 days a cycle cuts it to zero. However, adding progestogen causes most women on it to have a period-like bleed every month, and recent studies suggest progestogen may need to be taken only three or four times a year.

Hormone replacement therapy can be either oestrogen alone (called unopposed), or oestrogen plus progestogen (opposed), and can be given by mouth or applied as skin creams, skin patches, implants or vaginal creams or pessaries. Oral therapy is still the most widely used, but what is suitable for any individual depends on personal preference and side effects. Someone who finds that taking the oestrogen tablets makes her nauseous, for example, may do well with a skin patch, while other women may find the patches set up skin irritations. The patch is more expensive than tablets, but it more closely mimics the natural path of oestrogen through a menstruating body.

Current research seems to show that taking progestogen as well as oestrogen lowers a woman's risk of endometrial cancer, compared with women who take oestrogen alone or even take no HRT at all. Women who have had a hysterectomy no longer need progestogen to protect them from endometrial cancer. They need only oestrogen. Progestogen also seems to reduce problems with breast tenderness in some women taking HRT.

Some doctors favour HRT as soon as a peri-menopausal woman has the first flushes and sweats. Others advocate it as a treatment for troublesome osteoporosis for the over-70s. Some doctors favour using HRT for just two or three years, while others think that, once started, HRT should be continued for 20 years or more, and then discontinued gradually over several months to reduce the risk of the symptoms reappearing.

Whatever decisions you and your doctor make about these issues, if you decide to try HRT, informed counselling and careful clinical management increase the chances that, sooner or later, it will be a success for you. Not everyone can tolerate it, and you should report any side effects to your doctor.

Often, switching to a different form of HRT is all that is needed if the first form you try is not a success. For some women, however, deciding whether to stick with the therapy comes down to weighing up whether the benefits outweigh the side effects, which include the return of periods if they are on a regime of oestrogen and progesterone replacement.

For those whom HRT suits, the **benefits** can be:

- Relief from hot flushes, night sweats, vaginal dryness, painful intercourse and bladder problems, and this may have a knock-on effect on mood and mental well-being.

- Preventing or slowing bone loss. (Estimates of the reduced incidence of bone fractures resulting from HRT use range between 15 per cent and 50 per cent.)
- A probable reduction in the risk of heart disease and strokes, with the right type and strength of progestogen. (Some studies have put the reduction in the rate of untimely death in women on HRT from these causes as high as 50 per cent. But since doctors will prescribe HRT only to women who are already fairly healthy to start with, this factor along with class–related inequalities about HRT take-up may have skewed the results in HRT's favour.)
- A reduced risk of endometrial cancer if progestogen as well as oestrogen is taken (although this cancer kills fewer than 1400 women each year in England and Wales).
- Oestrogens (depending on the type and method of administration) can lower harmful LDL cholesterol and raise protective HDL (see p. 85).
- Increased life expectancy and enhanced quality of later life.

But the **drawbacks** can be:

- An increase to about one-and-a-half times the usual breast cancer risk if oestrogen is taken for more than 10 years. The danger may be greater for women with benign breast disease or whose mothers have had breast cancer, and progestogens may not reduce this risk.
- No firm finding yet on ovarian cancer. Studies have not so far found an increased risk in woman on HRT. However, there is a possible genetic link between cancers of the breast and ovaries, and more research is needed in this area.
- Progestogen can cancel out the beneficial effects on cholesterol of oestrogen alone (described above).
- Progestogen not only promotes the return of periods but can also bring back premenstrual syndrome, with bloating, mood swings and increased breast tenderness.

Research to improve HRT is continuing all the time. Meanwhile, whether to join the HRT club or not is not an option open to all. Some women try it, but decide on balance its side effects outweigh the actual or potential benefits. For others, if the results of one regime disappoint, they do better if they are switched to another. For still others, the decision can be complicated, or even completely ruled out, by other problems or conditions.

Diabetes might need re-stabilisation on HRT. Benign breast disease would need careful monitoring. Oestrogen can worsen gall bladder disease and endometriosis, and cause fibroids to become larger. Liver disease may, if it is severe enough, rule out HRT completely. Some conditions narrow the range of possible choices. Smoking, which increases the risk of heart and circulation problems, also accelerates the destruction of oestrogen and may therefore reduce the potential beneficial effects of HRT.

HRT is discussed in more detail in the Which? Consumer Guide *Understanding HRT and the Menopause*★★.

Help without HRT

If hormone replacement is not for you, there are other ways to minimise the effects of the peri-menopause and the menopause, and to maximise your health through the years of change. They include:

Diet It helps to eat as healthy a diet as you can to keep yourself well-nourished and your weight within sensible limits. The ingredients of a healthy diet and the availability and importance of calcium in avoiding osteoporosis are discussed in Chapter 3.

Keeping your blood sugar level fairly steady can help enormously, too. It is not difficult to see why. Symptoms of low blood sugar coincide with those some women suffer about the time they are going through the change anyway. They can include lack of energy and listlessness, sudden feelings of nervousness, forgetfulness and confusion, being anxious and worried for no apparent reason, periods of irritability, bouts of depression, and wanting to cry.

What happens is something like this. Our bodies break down carbohydrates into glucose for fuel, but when too much glucose is circulating in the body, the hormone insulin takes it out and stores it in the liver as glycogen. When we need more available fuel, the glycogen is converted back into glucose and released into the bloodstream again. When we eat too much sugar in a short space of time, the system goes into overdrive and ends up removing too much glucose, leaving our blood sugar level too low to get us comfortably to the next scheduled meal. Most of us know that limp-lettuce-leaf feeling that can set in during the late morning or late afternoon when we have gone some hours without food.

To avoid letting your blood sugar level fluctuate too much for comfort, don't go too long without eating something: better an apple or a banana sooner than a bag of crisps or a cream cake later. You may find you feel much better on a regular regime of four or five or even six small meals rather than three larger ones a day. Avoiding too much coffee, tea, alcohol and sugar, and too many processed foods, also helps.

Caffeine, alcohol, heavily spiced foods, hot drinks and sugar can be hot-flush triggers, too, so are best kept to a minimum or avoided altogether if you are experiencing these wild body-temperature swings – especially late in the day if you are having sleep problems and night sweats. The earlier you eat your evening meal and the lighter it is, the better and more comfortably you may find you sleep.

On a more positive note, some women find vitamins C and E helpful for hot flushes, and E for nervousness, fatigue, insomnia, dizziness, palpitations and shortness of breath. You may find you need as much as 400mg of vitamin E a day. Experiment and take the smallest supplementary dose that helps, allowing for the fact that it may take three or four weeks before you feel the benefit.

Many women find herbs, including sage, fenugreek, gotu kola, sarsaparilla, licorice root, wild yam root (which is the source for synthetic progestogens), ginseng and tan kawai (which is also known as female ginseng) helpful. Camomile and other herbal teas may also be relaxing.

(A helpful book for women who don't want or can't take HRT is *Menopause without Medicine*** by Linda Ojeda.)

Exercise It is hard to overstate the benefit of exercise for women around the time of the menopause. The importance of load-bearing exercise in fighting back against bone loss was explained in Chapter 2. Moreover, the stronger and more supple we remain, the less we are at risk of accidental fracture of thinner bones.

Equally important is the contribution that aerobic exercise can make to weight control, which also often becomes more of a problem for women from around 40 onwards. In addition, exercise is a potent mood enhancer, and can be enormously helpful for women whose response to the menopause is a bout of the blues. Some studies have even found it superior to anti-depressant drugs in alleviating depression. (There is more about dealing with the psychological problems that can occur around this time in a woman's life in Chapters 7 and 8.)

Life-style changes A number of small changes in one's life style may help minimise the unpleasant side effects of being peri-menopausal or menopausal. They include the following:

- Several layers of light clothing can be more comfortable than fewer heavier ones because they are more easily adaptable to how you feel from minute to minute.
- You may find natural fibres more comfortable to wear than synthetic ones.
- Lukewarm showers may be better for you than hot baths.
- If you are into serious night sweats, you may find it more comfortable if you put soft absorbent cotton towels over your sheets.
- Many smokers find the first puff of a cigarette often triggers a hot flush.
- It is worth checking with your doctor if you are on any medication as to whether it is likely to induce or exacerbate flushes.
- A milky drink at bedtime may help you sleep better. As menopausal women lose more calcium at night, a milky bedtime drink also helps to compensate for this.

The male menopause

We still have much to discover about whether there really is a male menopause, or climacteric, comparable with the changes that women's bodies go through, and if there is, exactly how and when it happens and how long it lasts.

Men in their middle years don't have the hot flushes and night sweats that plague these years for many women. But some men do complain of other symptoms reported by women – such as headaches, loss of memory, difficulty in making decisions, lack of energy and confidence, and tiredness and depression. Many men at this time of their lives also complain of a drop in sex drive and increasing difficulties in sexual performance, especially in regard to erection problems.

Outwardly at least, the middle and later years seem a time when little is happening to men compared with the rapid physiological response they experienced to the start of testosterone production by the testicles shortly before puberty. Fertility and production of the male sex hormone testosterone can persist into the 80s. If there is a hormonal mechanism at work in what is often referred to as a mid-life crisis, it may be produced not by testosterone reduction so much as by some still-undiscovered factor that is interfering with normal testosterone functioning.

Hormone treatment

The benefits of giving men testosterone to treat the symptoms of mid-life crisis, or even of making hormone replacement therapy as freely available to men as it is to women, are still disputed within the medical profession.

There is some evidence in favour. At the Hormonal Healthcare Centre in Harley Street, London, around 400 men between the ages of 30 and 80 have been treated with testosterone, and 80 per cent reported a moderate to a marked improvement in symptoms, including restoration to what they would have considered a normal sex drive a few years earlier.

But such treatment will remain controversial and unlikely to become generally available until it has been subjected to controlled clinical trials. Until testosterone therapy treatment passes such tests, it will be available only privately, and if you want to try it, you can expect it to cost you some hundreds of pounds for consultations, screening and treatment. (Screening is essential because of possible links between the treatment and prostate cancer.)

Masters and Johnson suggested as long ago as 1970 that men who find their sex drive declining in their middle years may be showing signs of lowered levels of male hormones, particularly testosterone. But they also attributed men's reduced sex desire around and beyond 40 to such non-hormonal causes as monotony in a long-running relationship, worry about money and jobs, the stress of going through what is probably the most competitive phase of their careers, mental and physical fatigue, and over-indulgence in food and alcohol.

Psychological factors

Modern sexologists would update that list with such particularly 1990s stresses as unemployment or fear of redundancy in an age when chances of finding another job decline sharply with age, and fear of sexually transmitted diseases such as herpes and particularly AIDS. Some men in today's youth culture mourn deeply the passing of their youthful looks, just as some women do. Some fret over the end of active parenthood when children leave home.

Rewriting traditional sexual and family roles has left some people unsure of what is expected of them in relationships or of their ability to deliver it. There are men who don't cope at all well when partners, who no longer are so handicapped by family responsibility, start new careers or begin to have real success in existing ones.

Although our understanding of the psychology of sexual diffi-culty may have been refined somewhat, the questions Masters and Johnson posed about the relative roles of hormones and psychology remain largely unanswered nearly a quarter of a century later.

Not only is it difficult, as it is with the female menopause, to tease apart physical and psychological factors, but it is also true that men who are unhappy with what they see as a decline in potency (whatever its actual causes) may respond in any one of a number of ways. Some try to prove they are still young by continually chasing younger women, or leaving home to settle in a new 'nest' with one. Some use prostitutes or rent boys. Some buy fast, expensive cars and splash out on clothes and cosmetic surgery. Others withdraw completely from sexual activity inside or outside marriage rather than risk being tried and perhaps found wanting. Some simply become depressed.

Some positive steps

If it is still uncertain whether men would benefit from having hormone replacement therapy as widely available to them as it now is to women, there are other steps they can take to help them to sail more comfortably through the middle years. These include:

- regular exercise (see above and Chapters 1 and 2)
- a healthy diet (as discussed in Chapter 3)
- not smoking, and drinking only in moderation (as discussed in Chapter 4)
- dealing sensibly and effectively with stress (see suggestions in Chapter 7)
- having an open and positive attitude towards change (discussed further in Chapter 8).

CHAPTER 6

KEEPING HEALTH PROBLEMS AT BAY

WE ALL HOPE to sail through our 40s and 50s and beyond feeling fit and healthy. But there are problems that become more likely to affect us as the decades pass. This chapter looks at some of them and at what may be helpful to know in dealing with them.

Health problems and self-help

Back trouble

Pain in the back is not an illness but a symptom, and can indicate a malfunction of the spine or its supporting musculature. The reason can be muscle strain, a trapped nerve, ankylosing spondy-litis (a chronic inflammatory condition or arthritis, predominantly affecting spinal joints) or any one of a dozen other causes. It can even be a symptom of kidney disease or gynaecological problems, or more serious problems like cancer attacking the bones of the spine.

More commonly, back pain is caused by excessive strain on the lower spine as a result of poor posture, being overweight, doing too much heavy lifting or lifting or carrying incorrectly.

Because the spine is such a complex piece of engineering (and one in some ways not well suited to a long life on two legs rather than four), the passage of time does it no favours. Degenerative change can start as early as our teens, but it becomes more likely later. As the years pass, the whole spine tends to become stiffer – lack of or incorrect exercise doesn't help – reducing the total range of movement. Tissues in the spine also become stiffer and less ready to change shape, reducing their ability to absorb shock. In this way, degeneration can affect the whole spine or just a single site.

Because back problems can be caused by violent injury or gradual deterioration, or by disease which does not necessarily involve the spine at all, it can be difficult to diagnose the precise cause of back pain. As a result, people who complain of back ache are sometimes unjustly accused of malingering, and treatment can be problematical, too. Back pain has an added sting in the tail: once you have had it, the more likely it is that you will get it again. Most back pain, in fact, clears up with bed-rest and painkillers even before detailed investigations are carried out, so the cause often is never known. But if it persists after 48 hours of lying flat, you should see a doctor.

Self-help

Regular exercise – swimming, for example – is important for people who suffer with back problems, but it should be subject to some special precautions. These are outlined in Chapter 1 and given in more detail in the Which? Consumer Guide *Understanding Back Trouble***, which also contains exercises designed specifically to strengthen different parts of the back.

Protecting your back involves not carrying around heavy things – including excessive body weight – sitting correctly when you are working and having desk and equipment appropriately positioned. It means squatting rather than bending and knowing how to lift, shift and carry correctly. To lift a load, make sure you are as close to it as possible and stand so you are firmly balanced. Bend the hips and knees, grasp the load firmly – and straighten the back so it is in the line of gravity and so that leg muscles rather than back muscles are doing the lifting.

Sitting properly means doing so in a chair where your feet are flat on the ground and knees are level with or slightly above your hips. The seat should support three-quarters of the backs of your thighs and should not dig in behind your knees. Work surfaces should be at elbow height. A pamphlet called *Are you sitting comfortably?* is available free (but send an s.a.e.) from the Arthritis and Rheumatism Council*, and describes what to look for when you are choosing an easy chair.

TECHNIQUE OF LIFTING

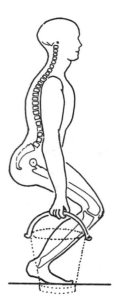

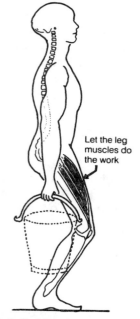

Let the leg muscles do the work

1. Squat, rather than stoop, to grasp the load

2. Straighten the back so that it is in the line of gravity, then let the leg muscles do the lifting

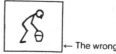
← The wrong way to lift!

Cancer

Cancer is not one specific disease; there are more than 100 varieties of it. What they all have in common is an unrestrained growth of cells inside a specific organ or tissue of the body. In short, cancer is normal cell division gone haywire. However, many cancers grow more slowly the older we are, so increasing the chances of successful treatment if the disease is detected early enough.

The older we are, the more likely we are to develop cancers of the skin, lungs and digestive tract, and several forms of leukaemia. The chance of women developing breast cancer increases somewhat, and of men developing cancer of the prostate much more sharply, with age.

Cancer of the cervix (neck of the womb) has a more complex pattern. Risk of it rises steeply from the mid-20s to the mid-40s, falls off slightly for a few years, then reaches an even higher peak from age 65 to 75. The risk of cancer of the uterus (the womb itself) rises sharply from 40 onwards, and also doesn't peak until around the age of 75.

Self-help

Prevention There is increasing evidence of links between our diet and the likelihood that we will suffer cancer. Eating too much fat is suspected of increasing the risk of breast, colon and prostate cancers (though this evidence is as yet inconclusive). Cancers of the uterus, gall bladder and breast are all believed to be obesity-related.

One of the more exciting developments in nutrition in recent years has been the increasing awareness of the effect of the antioxidants beta-carotene, which is a precursor of vitamin A, and vitamins C and E, plus the mineral selenium. They seem to offer some protection from cancers and heart disease. Their role is explained in detail in Chapter 3. Fruit and vegetables are the main sources of the antioxidant vitamins; hence the importance of at least five portions a day now recommended as a healthy diet. Selenium can be found in meat, especially kidneys, brazil nuts, oily fish and bread. A diet high in fibre is also important, particularly in the prevention of cancer of the colon.

Smoking increases the risk of lung cancer and some other cancers, including leukaemia and cancers of the lip, mouth, nose, throat, larynx, oesophagus, cervix, kidney, bladder and pancreas.

Taking oestrogen-only hormone replacement therapy (HRT) for more than 10 years increases the risk of breast cancer to about one-and-a-half times the average. The risk may be greater for women with benign breast disease or whose mothers have had breast cancer than for others. Oestrogen-only HRT also increases the likelihood in women who have not had a hysterectomy of hyperplasia, the thickening of the lining of the uterus that can be a forerunner of endometrial cancer.

Current research in the US, however, seems to show that taking both progestogen and oestrogen (rather than just oestrogen) lowers the risk of endometrial cancer to less than it is even for women the same age not using HRT at all. (HRT also seems to offer protection against heart disease and osteoporosis, discussed below.)

Avoiding excessive exposure to sunlight is important in preventing all three types of skin cancer, which are becoming increasingly prevalent in the UK. Around 40,000 new cases of skin cancer are diagnosed in the country every year, and the number is on the increase. Perhaps even more worryingly, the rarest but most dangerous of the three types of skin cancer – malignant melanoma – is also on the rise. There were 1300 deaths from it in Britain in 1993.

It is important to wear a hat and avoid sunbathing between 11am and 3pm if you are in a hot country and between noon and 2pm in the UK. Use a sunscreen and reapply it after sweating heavily or after a couple of hours in the sun. When you are swimming, make sure you go for water-resistant versions of sunscreen and remember that you will still need to reapply it as soon as you come out of the water.

If you have fair skin and freckles (or had freckles as a child), you are in the group at greatest risk. You should wear a sunscreen with a sun protection factor (SPF) of 15 for at least your first six days in the heat, and if you are really wise, stick with it even after that. In any case, it is better for you never to go down to less than about factor 8. People who tan more readily may want to start reducing the numbers after about four days, but even they should never go below 6.

In addition, make sure your sunscreen is formulated to work against both UVA and UVB rays. As well as an overall SPF number, many products now also have a UVA rating of 1, 2, 3 or 4 stars, with 1 being only moderate and 4 maximum.

Exposure to the sun not only poses a skin-cancer risk, but also causes premature ageing of skin. The good news, however, is that products to turn the skin brown without sun are getting better all the time. More and more people are asking themselves, why burn – or worse – for it when you can fake it?

Some medical authorities believe stress is also a factor in cancers.

Detection One of the most powerful self-help measures for cancer is early detection so that medical treatment can start as soon as possible. That means that all women who are, or have been, sexually active should have regular cervical smear tests, ideally every year to the age of 65 and every two or three years thereafter. At the moment, the NHS routinely offers a smear only once every three years, so if you want one more often you will probably have to pay, unless you are at a higher-than-average risk for some reason.

It is also important to practise regular self-examination for lumps or thickening anywhere in the breasts. Ideally, this should be done during the first few days after the menstrual period for pre-menopausal women and on a regular date, such as the first of the month, for women who no longer menstruate.

Changes that you should take notice of are:

- any difference in the size of a breast
- if one breast has become lower than the other
- a lump or lumpy area
- if the position of a nipple has changed, or a nipple is turning in
- a nipple discharging liquid
- a skin rash or change of skin texture or colour
- enlarged glands in the armpits or above or below the collar-bones
- a swelling of the upper arm.

Mammograms may cause brief discomfort, but this is worth enduring. They involve 'squashing' the breast between two plates in order to get an X-ray picture of the breast tissue. This breast X-ray technique can detect cancers so small they cannot be felt by examination.

Opinion both sides of the Atlantic is divided over the age at which regular breast screening should start. Some organisations advocate as early as between 35 and 40, others not until 50 and beyond. Research in the UK has so far been inconclusive; a major study is currently being conducted, but the results are years away.

At the moment, the NHS is offering screening free every three years to all women between 50 and 64, and women over 64 who request it will also be included in the programme. But one in five breast cancer deaths now occur before 55, and screening only from 50 onwards will do little to reduce that figure. Screening every three years may mean nearly as many cancers will be missed as found once regular screening does start. So it is still important for women to practise regular self-examination and go to the doctor if they find anything, no matter how small, that wasn't there last time.

At least one private health screening organisation advocates women start at 40 and are screened every year. It is quite possible that the NHS will change to offering mammography to younger women and more frequently.

There has been some concern about the safety of mammography because of the danger of regular exposure to radiation. In fact, the test subjects a women to no more risk of radiation-induced breast cancer than does smoking a quarter of a cigarette a day.

Although testicular cancer occurs most frequently in men aged between 20 and 35, older men should still practise regular testicle self-examination. Treatment of testicular cancer, if found early, is a success story. The treatment is extremely unpleasant, but the outcome is very good indeed.

To do your regular self-examination, you need to be aware of how your testicles usually feel so you can spot any change in size, shape or firmness and see a doctor about it. The best time to do it is after a warm bath or shower because the scrotal skin is loose and relaxed then. What you need to do is support your scrotum and testicles in the palm of one hand to check their size and weight. Then gently roll first one and then the other testicle between the thumb and the index and middle fingers of the other hand.

How to look
Undressed to the waist, sit in front of a mirror in good light.

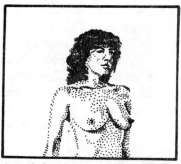

1. Look: hands at your sides or on your hips, look carefully at your breasts. Turn from side to side. Look underneath too.

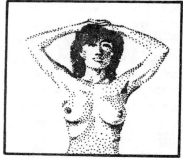

2. Lift: hands on your head, look for anything unusual, especially around the nipple.

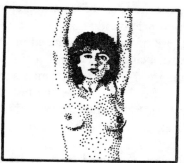

3. Stretch: arms stretched above your head, look again, particularly around the nipple.

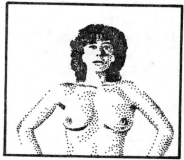

4. Press: hands on hips, press inwards until your chest muscles tighten. Look again, especially for any dimpling of the skin.

BREAST EXAMINATION

How to feel
Lie on a flat surface, head on a pillow, shoulder slightly raised by a folded towel.

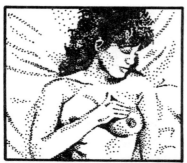

5. Left shoulder raised, feel the left breast with the right hand. Use the flat of the fingers, keeping them together.

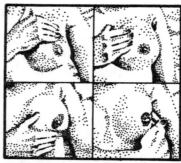

6. Press the breast gently but firmly in towards the body. Work in a spiral, circling out from the nipple. Feel every part.

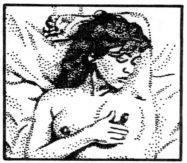

7. Left arm above your head, elbow bent, repeat the spiral carefully. Feel the outer part of the breast especially.

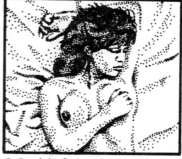

8. Finish by feeling the tail of the breast towards the armpit. Repeat all four stages on the other breast. Be thorough. Don't rush.

By kind permission of the Women's Nationwide Cancer Control Campaign.

For both men and women, there are a number of other symptoms that you should also report to your doctor. They probably aren't but could just possibly be cancer warnings. They are:

- change of bowel or bladder habits
- blood in urine or faeces
- abdominal pain that persists or recurs
- unexplained and sudden weight loss
- a change of voice
- a sore that does not heal
- unusual bleeding or discharge
- thickening or lump in the breast or elsewhere in the body
- obvious change of shape, size or colour in a mole or wart
- nagging cough or hoarseness
- breathlessness
- a headache you can't seem to get rid of or that often recurs
- any scab, sore or ulcer that does not heal in three weeks
- a persistent white patch inside the mouth
- chest pains.

Some people put off going to the doctor when they fear the diagnosis will be cancer. By delaying because of what they fear they might hear, they could be allowing a disease to take hold or worrying unnecessarily about a perfectly innocent condition. More cancers are being treated more successfully every year, and the earlier treatment starts, the better the chance of success. The importance of early investigation cannot be overemphasised.

Exercise, with its beneficial effects on both physical and mental well-being, can be an important self-help element in recovery after surgery or other treatments for cancer. Discuss with your doctor how soon, how much and what type would help you best.

Heart disease

Heart disease is something of a misnomer, as the problems associated with this general term are not actually diseases of the heart but defects in the system by which oxygenated blood is supplied to the heart.

Men can suffer serious heart disease as early as their 30s or 40s. Women seem to gain some protection from oestrogen until the menopause, after which heart disease rates rise – although hormone replacement therapy (see Chapter 5) seems partly to restore protection for as long as women are having it. Pre-menopausal women most at risk are smokers aged 35 and over who are on the contraceptive pill.

Women have been conspicuously underrepresented in major studies of risk factors for heart disease in both the US and Britain. Most studies have concentrated on men only, while a few have looked at both. No major study has as yet focused on women alone and, as far as we know, risk factors for women mirror those of men. The omission of women from the research is the more remarkable when you realise that, in the UK, coronary heart disease is the second largest cause (after cancer) of premature death in women under 65 and the main cause after 65 – by which time the rate is almost the same as for men of the same age.

Recent British studies have found that men are one-and-a-half times more likely to be offered surgery for heart disease than are women, and that if women go to their doctors complaining of symptoms of chest pain, breathlessness and palpitations, they are less likely to be referred to heart specialists than are men with the same symptoms. To date, operations done on women for heart disease have also tended to be less successful, and the difference has been put down to the fact that their smaller hearts and arteries make them more difficult for surgeons to work on.

However true that may be, it must now be considered at least open to question whether this accounts for all the discrepancy. If there is a greater reluctance to refer women to specialists and to offer surgery, could it be that those who do get to undergo operations are more seriously ill than men, on average, by the time they reach the operating table?

The stereotypical heart-disease victim is an overweight busi-nessman in a stressful, probably deskbound job who gets too little exercise and eats too 'well'. Like most stereotypes it contains a grain of truth. Being overweight, getting too little exercise, being under too much stress and having too rich a diet are all known risk factors for men. But men and women from all walks of life die of heart disease.

The three main types of heart disease are angina, heart attacks and heart-valve disease.

Angina This is cramp of the heart muscle caused when too little oxygen and nutrients are reaching it, usually because the coronary arteries which supply the heart have become clogged with fatty deposits. This condition is called atherosclerosis. The symptoms of angina – pain varying from a mild aching to a crushing sensation or tightness across the centre of the chest, sometimes spreading to neck, jaw or arms – are similar to those of a heart attack. Angina usually comes on with exertion and eases off after a few minutes of resting. (A heart attack, by contrast, can last several hours and if not treated can cause permanent damage to the heart muscle – see below.)

An electrocardiogram (ECG) to record the electrical activity passing through the heart muscle is usually done to confirm a diagnosis of angina. Treatment can include drugs to widen the coronary arteries and reduce the heart's demand for oxygen by slowing it down. Surgery may be necessary for some angina sufferers. Techniques include angioplasty, in which a balloon is inflated inside narrowed arteries to flatten the fatty deposits, and bypass surgery, in which an artery from the leg is grafted into the chest to bypass the blockage or blockages.

Heart attacks These can occur when one or more arteries becomes so narrow that a clot can actually block off the blood supply completely and the starved heart muscle begins to die. The extent of the damage and the intensity of the pain of a heart attack depends on exactly where the blockage is. If it is quite near the bottom of the heart, in one of the smaller arteries, only a small section of heart muscle will be damaged. The heart may even grow new small arteries to bypass the blocked artery in time. But if the blockage is near the origin of one of the three main coronary arteries, then a terrible crushing pain can spread from the chest to the neck and arms, and the heart attack can be fatal. (If the blood supply to the brain is blocked, the result is a stroke; see below.)

Sudden death after a heart attack can sometimes be caused not by the blockage itself but by a complication that follows it. When a large part of the muscle dies, the natural rhythm can be disturbed, and instead of beating regularly, the ventricles can start to quiver or flutter. This can be fatal because it means that no blood is being pumped around the body to vital organs such as the brain and the heart. Machines called defibrillators can literally shock the heart back into beating rhythmically, but only if they can be used very quickly. All hospitals have them, and so do some ambulances and general practitioners' surgeries.

Heart-valve disease This is caused when something goes wrong with one of the four heart valves and the heart's ability to pump blood effectively is reduced. Fortunately, heart-valve problems can usually be put right fairly simply by replacing or repairing the problem valve.

You may like to know that there is a Which? Consumer Guide called *Preventing Heart Disease*★★, which discusses the heart and heart problems in greater detail.

Self-help

Too high a level of saturates in our diet and cholesterol in our blood increases the risk of heart disease. The complex relationship between cholesterol and saturates intake in the build-up of dangerous fatty deposits in arteries is explained in Chapter 3. One way to reduce the risk of heart disease is to stick to a diet rich in fruit and vegetables – also discussed in Chapter 3, and in the section on cancer, above.

Lack of exercise (see Chapters 1 and 2), smoking and immoderate drinking (discussed in Chapter 4) are risk factors for heart disease. In fact, some hospitals are now reluctant to do bypass operations on smokers, because they say continuing to smoke reduces the likelihood of success. Unless one makes life-style changes, including eating a healthier diet, taking off excess weight and having more exercise, surgery may in any case bring only a temporary relief. Arteries widened by angioplasty or grafts that have replaced clogged arteries can fur up all over again if they are subjected to the same life style.

A return to exercise or even starting to exercise for the first time after a heart attack or surgery can help speed recovery as well as helping to prevent a recurrence. But exercise will need to be taken gently and built up gradually. Start only when and at the rate your specialist says it is safe for you.

Some studies have shown that small daily doses of aspirin (one-quarter to one-half soluble tablet) can reduce the risk of having another heart attack, although this may not be suitable for people who suffer stomach upsets or other side effects from aspirin. Aspirin can also interfere with other drugs prescribed for coronary heart disease. So check with your doctor first before deciding on whether aspirin is right for you.

HRT seems to give women some protection against heart disease. Some studies have put the reduction as high as 50 per cent, although that figure is probably overoptimistic.

Self-help for all heart-disease sufferers, whether they are on drug therapy alone or they are post-surgery, also needs to include good stress management and relaxation techniques (see Chapter 7).

High blood pressure

Blood pressure is the pressure at which the heart pushes blood round the arteries of the body, and is influenced both by the force generated by the heart and by the elasticity of the arteries. When blood pressure is measured, the result is given as two different figures. The higher figure is the systolic pressure and is the reading at the moment the heart beats to expel blood, sending it on its way round the body, and expanding the walls of the arteries slightly as it goes. The lower figure, the diastolic pressure, is measured between beats when the heart muscle is at rest. It measures the pressure when the arteries, which expand slightly under the pressure of blood flowing out through them, ping back into shape like a slightly stretched rubber band. The more elasticity the artery walls retain, the healthier they are.

Both systolic and diastolic pressures are measured in millimetres of mercury. The convention is to write the systolic followed by the diastolic pressure thus: a systolic pressure of 140 and a diastolic pressure of 90 is written as 140/90.

Hypertension, or unhealthily high blood pressure, is often described as the silent killer because it creeps up without symptoms and, undetected and untreated, can cause extremely serious damage. Unless hypertension is discovered in a routine medical examination and treated, it can rupture an artery in the brain to leave a person paralysed and unable to speak after a stroke. High blood pressure increases the likelihood not only of a stroke but also of a number of other illnesses, including heart attack, heart failure, kidney disease and loss of sight following haemorrhage in the retina at the back of the eye.

What is too high is both age-related and culturally defined. A young person with a reading of more than 140/90 would be watched carefully, for fear that his or her condition might become serious over time. If someone had that reading at the age of 70, it would not be a cause for concern, however.

Even if blood pressure is healthy when a person is young, high blood pressure becomes increasingly likely with increasing age because the arteries become less elastic (as, for example, does a well-used rubber band). They are also narrowed by the build-up of deposits of fat (atherosclerosis, described under heart disease, above).

In the US, anything over 160/90 may be considered a suitable case for treatment with medication, while in Britain many doctors regard 200/120 as the critical point. What complicates the decision is that medication for blood pressure, though much improved now, can have side effects and overtreatment can actually be harmful. As yet, evidence of the effects on mortality when medication is introduced at different levels is scant and inconclusive.

One seven-year study in the US compared the effects of giving patients with an average blood pressure of 183/100 medication or a placebo. At the end of the study, 8 per cent of the drug-treated group and 11 per cent of the control group had died of a stroke or a heart attack, and the active treatment group also had had fewer non-fatal strokes and serious heart failures. Overall mortality was no different, however, for the two groups. Those who might have been spared a stroke or fatal heart attack by hypertension medication seemed to have died of something else anyway.

A further complication for doctors assessing treatments for raised blood pressure is that the anxiety of attending a surgery to have it taken possibly elevates an individual's blood pressure. Some doctors make it a rule to obtain the same high reading at least three times before they accept it as worth acting on.

Self-help
Make sure you have your blood pressure checked by your doctor or practice nurse at regular intervals, at least once every five years up to the age of about 50 or so and at least once a year if you are over 55.

Whatever a hypertension sufferer's doctor decides about drug therapy, there are a number of steps you can take to help yourself to stave off high blood pressure, or to lower it if it is already high. Even if yours is seriously enough elevated to require medication, self-help can assist by keeping the drug dose to a minimum.

A study reported in the *Journal of the American Medical Association* in March 1992 found that overweight patients who managed to lose around 9lbs in weight brought their blood pressure down comfortably by as much as 10mm of mercury. This means eating healthily and exercising regularly to get and keep excess weight off. Exercise has a direct effect on blood pressure as well, and is an aid to stress management, another vital component of self-help for those with high blood pressure. Relaxation techniques used regularly can help (see Chapter 7 on dealing with stress), and alcohol and caffeine intakes need to be lowered to acceptable levels.

The study mentioned above also found that cutting down on salt – the standard treatment for high blood pressure before the development of modern hypertension medication – also helped reduce it, but didn't make as much difference as losing excess body weight. It is also important not to smoke if you have high blood pressure. Smoking magnifies enormously the danger that hypertension will result in stroke or serious heart attack. There are tips on giving up smoking and reducing alcohol and caffeine intakes in Chapter 4.

Insomnia

Insomnia can include having difficulty getting to sleep or staying asleep, waking too early, or sleeping restlessly and waking still tired. There is no right amount of sleep. Some people feel wonderful on five hours a night and others don't sparkle on less than ten. And if you cannot get off to sleep, it is as well to remember that just lying in bed is doing you some good.

If sleep problems reflect stress in your life, the only cure for the symptom may be to sort out the cause. The next chapter is devoted to the subject of discovering sources of stress and eliminating or reducing them.

Self-help

There are self-help measures for insomnia given under the heading Sleep problems in the next chapter.

Obesity

Obesity, its dangers and how to measure and deal with it are all discussed under the heading How much is too much? in Chapter 3.

Osteoarthritis

Osteoarthritis is the most common form of arthritis and is caused by wear and tear of the cartilage surfaces inside a joint. This causes pain, stiffness and swelling. Although more common after the age of 50, it can set in earlier, especially in the wake of injury. Osteoarthritis usually does not affect the whole body but is confined to one or two joints alone. It is not reversible, but that does not mean nothing can be done to ease the symptoms and slow down its progress.

Heavy manual labour can produce arthritis of the spine, hips, knees and ankles, and repetitive movements can cause it in the extremities – for example, 'ticket collector's thumb'. Osteoarthritis is likely to crop up in any joint that has suffered traumatic injury or has been damaged by overuse in playing sport.

Medical treatment is likely to be by painkilling or anti-inflammatory drugs taken orally or as a gel applied to the affected area. In severe cases, surgery may be indicated. Joint replacement surgery (most often for the hip) has given a new lease of life to tens of thousands of people. Surgery can also be used to do repair work on arthritic joints and to remove debris from within the joint space. Once a need for joint replacement has been indicated, the operation should be done sooner rather than later. Waiting only means enduring pain longer than necessary and increases the danger that some other condition may intervene to make surgery more difficult.

Waiting lists for hip replacements can be anything up to two years, and that is after you have waited for an initial consultation with a surgeon to establish suitability. So it is advisable to ask your doctor to set the wheels in motion as early as possible for you, while medication is holding symptoms in check.

The hip operation involves replacing the ball joint at the top of the femur with one made of cobalt. People who have it need crutches for the first six to twelve weeks out of hospital, and take about another month or two to get back to normal walking.

Self-help

Carrying excess body weight aggravates osteoarthritis. Every extra pound increases the strain on arthritic joints.

Regular exercise that does not involve putting weight on load-bearing joints – swimming, cycling and so on – helps. So do stretching exercises that put joints gently through their full range of movements. Your doctor or a physiotherapist (see p.162) can help you with advice on what you should avoid and what is right for you.

Specific exercises to strengthen muscles around an arthritic joint can also help by ensuring the muscles do not waste from underuse and by protecting the joint against further damage. A physiotherapist can help advise you as to exactly what is needed. Some people find applying heat packs helpful, and it is important to warm up affected joints before exercise and avoid extreme cold even when warmly dressed.

Some osteoarthritis sufferers find manipulative therapies such as osteopathy, chiropractic or physiotherapy helpful, too. Details of how to find qualified practitioners are given at the end of this chapter.

It is also particularly important for osteoarthritis sufferers to follow the advice on lifting correctly given in the section on Back trouble, above. Good posture is important, and so is wearing properly fitted shoes. Rest can also be good therapy. There are a number of aids available to make life easier by taking pressure off affected joints while doing everyday chores. For example, self-opening scissors with larger-than-average loops will comfortably accommodate swollen fingers.

Osteoporosis

Osteoporosis is the thinning of bones which become honeycombed by loss of collagen and calcium over time. Bone mass is reduced so that bone breaks more easily, especially at the hips, wrists and spine.

One woman in ten can expect to have a hip fracture between the ages of 70 and 75. And for between one in ten and one in five of them it will be fatal. Between a quarter and half of the rest will never regain the level of functioning they had before it.

Although women are more prone to it, men who live long enough may develop osteoporosis, too. Besides being more at risk of broken bones, sufferers may become shorter and develop the curvature of the spine called dowager's hump.

Self-help

The role of diet in the prevention and treatment of osteoporosis is discussed under the heading Brittle bones in Chapter 3. There is also advice on the most suitable forms of exercise to prevent osteoporosis and the safest exercises for people who have developed it in Chapter 2.

Hormone replacement therapy (HRT), discussed in Chapter 5, seems to prevent the loss of bone calcium that causes the disease as long as the therapy is being taken, and to slow the rate of loss even after it is stopped. Some studies have suggested that when a woman takes HRT she makes it 50 per cent less likely that she will have an osteoporosis-related fracture in her lifetime, although other researchers dispute these findings as optimistically high.

Rheumatoid arthritis

Rheumatoid arthritis is one of the more disabling forms of arthritis and it can start at any age, but usually first appears in the 30s and 40s. It can start slowly or abruptly, even explosively. There are about three times as many women as men among the one million affected people in the UK. Its exact cause is unknown, but it is possibly one of the auto-immune diseases, in which the body's immune system starts to attack its own tissues. It is possibly precipitated by a virus.

The most frequently affected areas are the knees, hands, feet, neck and ankles, although the disease can appear in any joint and can also affect other organs. It can produce symptoms throughout the body, starting with tiredness, feverishness or weakness in the early stages, with possible loss of appetite and weight loss. Other indications might be inflamed eyes, pleurisy, lumps under the skin and inflammation of heart muscle, blood vessels and other tissues.

Some people have one severe attack and then remain symptom-free for a long period, although the symptoms usually reappear eventually. Sufferers may have alternating flare-ups and remissions lasting years for the rest of their lives. Rheumatoid arthritis can cause stiffness, making joint movements both difficult and painful. Unchecked, bones may fuse completely, which may eradicate pain but will result in loss of joint function.

Early diagnosis and treatment minimise damage. Medication, as well as exercise and other treatments, can help maintain joint mobility. At a later stage, the only effective way to correct a serious deformity or improve the range of movement in a joint or joint replacement may be surgery. As well as artificial hips, there are artificial joints for knees, fingers and shoulders which can replace joints that have become very stiff or uncomfortable.

Self-help
People with rheumatoid arthritis need to organise their time to include periods of rest and exercise which will help maintain mobility. Both need to be done in moderation and exercise should be done every day, except during a flare-up of particu-larly hot, painful joints (when applying cold packs may give relief).

Applying heat or having a warm bath before exercise can be helpful, as can gentle stretching to warm up the body. It is important to put each joint in the body through its full range of movement each day. Swimming, especially in a warm pool, is good therapy. Short exercise periods several times a day are better than one long session.

Regular sessions of physiotherapy between flare-ups can loosen up the joints and strengthen the muscles that support them. Acupuncture may help with pain relief. There are a variety of aids, such as those mentioned under the section on Osteoarthritis, above, which can also be helpful for everyday chores such as preparing food and dressing.

Stroke

A stroke follows the interruption of normal blood supply to part of the brain and the consequent damage of cells deprived of oxygen for more than a few minutes. Strokes become more likely with age; half of them occur in people over 75, and men are at higher risk than women.

Strokes are usually one of three main kinds. They can be a cerebral thrombosis, caused by a blood clot obstructing one of the main arteries of the brain; a cerebral embolism, where a broken-off fragment of blood clot blocks a brain artery; and a cerebral haemorrhage, where a blood vessel in the brain ruptures.

The symptoms following a stroke depend largely on the part of the brain that is damaged by it. Each brain area controls specific functions in particular parts of the body. Thus there may be numbness or weakness on one side of the body, loss or slurring of speech, partial loss of vision, dizziness, confusion, a fall or unconsciousness, or a sudden severe headache. Diagnosis will only be confirmed after a thorough physical examination, and the extent of damage may be assessed by one of a number of brain-imaging techniques.

Surgery is not usually required after a stroke. Treatment is more likely to be drugs to dissolve a clot or prevent it enlarging or to keep further clots from developing. Rehabilitation after a stroke involves a programme to improve physical abilities and restore independence. Damaged nerve tissue cannot regenerate, but other parts of the brain may, with training, learn to take over the functions of the damaged area.

Self-help

Prevention measures include not smoking, keeping drinking to moderate levels, taking regular exercise, eating a low-fat, high-fibre diet, and watching your weight. Regular blood pressure checks are also essential, since raised blood pressure is an early warning of possible strokes.

It is also important to tell you doctor if you have had a transient ischaemic attack (TIA), or mini-stroke. You could have had one if you have experienced any of these symptoms:

- sudden blackout
- temporary loss of speech or vision
- brief, unexplained loss of power or sensation in an arm or leg.

Symptoms will disappear completely within 24 hours and leave no disability, but they can be an early warning of an approaching stroke. Just how early is variable; many strokes are preceded by a mini-stroke anything from a few days to several months before. So if you experience any of these symptoms, seek assessment without delay.

Taking aspirin regularly may help to prevent another stroke. (But see the section on Heart attacks, above, for information about the dose – and a caution.)

The special role of exercise

Exercise has a three-fold contribution to make to good health. First is its major role in disease prevention, as already discussed in Chapter 1. Second, exercise can also be an important self-help measure in treating many conditions. For people with hypertension, for example, exercise can be a way of avoiding having to take medication, or of minimising the amount of medication needed.

Third, it can have a psychological benefit which can have a knock-on physical effect on a wide range of conditions. People feel better when they exercise, and both the physical and psychological benefits of exercise can help recovery after surgery and other treatments for many conditions, including cancers and heart problems.

Recognition of the role of exercise in treating as well as preventing ill health is becoming more widespread in the medical profession. There are now around 150 practices in the country where the doctors have an arrangement with a local health club or leisure centre, to which they 'prescribe' patients with a variety of conditions to go for a course of exercise as part of their treatment.

If your doctor does not have such a scheme, you could still ask him or her about the advisability of exercise for you, and what will most help you and what you should avoid.

Alternative paths to self-help

Many people, including a number of doctors, no longer believe conventional medicine has all the answers to every health problem. Some other approaches are discussed below.

Chiropractic

Chiropractic was developed in the West around the turn of the century by an American, David D. Palmer. A caretaker in the building where he worked had become deaf when he bent over awkwardly and felt something give way in his back. Years later, Palmer located the spot, put the misaligned vertebra back into place and restored the man's hearing.

Palmer spent the rest of his life researching and seeking recognition for the therapy that he developed following that dramatic debut, based on the idea that most of what goes wrong with joints and bones is caused by incorrect alignment of the vertebrae. His theory was that the spine presses on nerves and causes problems in the rest of the body.

Although they began from different theoretical positions, there are similarities today between chiropractic and osteopathic techniques and approach (see below), including the fact that both chiropractors and osteopaths regard the body as essentially self-healing. They see their role as freeing trapped nerve tissue so the body can get on with making itself healthy again.

Osteopaths tend to work more on muscles and tendons and use leverage, while chiropractors tend to use direct pressure on the affected areas. Chiropractors are more likely to use X-rays and other diagnostic tests than osteopaths, though some osteopaths use them too. Today, there is also considerable overlap between the therapies, and many practitioners of both regard their theoretical differences as mostly historical.

Chiropractors take full case histories with details of life style as well as of past and present health, usually before they start a physical examination. They will often give life-style advice. Chiropractors deal with back problems and neck pain, stiffness, migraine, catarrh, sinusitis, digestive problems and menstrual problems, among others.

There have been six different government enquiries into chiropractic worldwide over the last 20 years, and each has concluded that its modern practice is safe when it is done by someone adequately trained.

A study funded by the British Medical Research Council compared the effectiveness of chiropractic and hospital out-patient treatment of low-back pain and actually found chiropractic treatment gave results that were better and lasted longer.

A chiropractor who has taken a four-year full-time training course that meets the internally recognised standard can become a member of the British Chiropractic Association★ and join its register.

Homoeopathy

Thousands of British doctors have now also trained in homoeopathy, and the numbers are growing every year. Some are attracted to it because they are unhappy about side effects of conventional or allopathic treatments and the extent to which they find themselves treating these side effects rather than the symptoms of the original problem.

Another appeal of the homoeopathic approach to its doctor and lay practitioners and to patients who seek it out is its ethos of treating the whole person and the underlying causes of illness rather than just the symptoms of a pathological condition. The system is based on the principle of treating like with like. It was founded by Dr Samuel Hahnemann, an eighteenth-century German physician and chemist who noticed that quinine was used to treat symptoms similar to those it would cause in a healthy body.

Hahnemann had already become disillusioned with particularly harsh and distressing contemporary treatments such as bleeding, purging and surgical operations done without anaesthetic or with much in the way of hygiene. He devoted the rest of his working life to finding other substances which had effects that were similar to those of quinine. Hahnemann believed illness results from the body being out of balance and that the physician's job is essentially to help it use its intrinsic and individual ability to heal itself.

Modern medicine increasingly attacks symptoms either by

blocking natural pathways in the body or by attacking the germs directly. Homoeopathy, on the other hand, sees symptoms as evidence that the body is at work on the job of healing itself. The system uses minute doses of substances that in larger quantities could cause in a healthy person the symptoms a patient is suffering. With this approach, symptoms may increase in severity before they begin to diminish.

Devoted followers include the Royal Family, and there are homoeopathic doctors and a small number of homoeopathic hospitals operating within the NHS.

If you go to a homoeopathic practitioner, the first consultation could well last more than an hour. He or she will want to build up a detailed picture of you and your feelings, family life, personality, likes and dislikes, as well as the particular symptom or symptoms troubling you. Treatments are decided both on the basis of what you are suffering and the type of person you are.

Write to the British Homoeopathic Association* for a doctor who is qualified in homoeopathy, or the Society of Homoeopaths* for a qualified lay homoeopath.

Osteopathy

Osteopathy focuses on the structure of the body and has in common with homoeopathy an underlying belief in the body's ability to heal itself. Again, as with homoeopathy, some doctors now also have training in osteopathy.

Its founder was another American, Andrew Taylor Still, who at the end of the last century became disillusioned with the shortcomings of conventional treatments of the day and felt that understanding how the body's structure relates to its use is the way to understand how health breaks down. He maintained that when the structure is misaligned, disease is caused.

Osteopathy also has a holistic philosophy. It sees patients as whole and individual people. Like chiropractors, osteopaths take full case histories which include not only details of present symptoms but also of an individual's record of illness and injury. Again like chiropractors, they will ask about life style, stress, exercise and so on before they begin to examine a patient. Treatment can be soft-tissue massage or manipulation, and can be gentle or quite firm.

Although many people think of osteopathy and back problems as almost synonymous, osteopaths also treat many other conditions, including rheumatism, arthritis, migraine, tension headaches, bronchitis, menstrual and even sexual and fertility problems.

Many organisations provide courses in osteopathy of varying length and content. The British School of Osteopathy, the European School of Osteopathy and the British College of Naturopathy and Osteopathy all run four-year full-time degree and diploma courses for people without medical qualifications. The London College of Osteopathic Medicine does a one-year course for doctors.

All these courses qualify people to call themselves registered osteopaths, to become members of the General Council and Register of Osteopaths★ and to use the initials MRO after their names. An osteopath using only the initials 'DO' may have nothing more than a diploma obtained by doing a correspondence course.

Physiotherapy

This is not so much an alternative therapy as an adjunct to conventional treatment, though as with osteopathy and chiropractic you can self-refer, and many people do when they are seeking relief from pain or to speed up healing or recovery.

Physiotherapists treat spinal problems such as slipped discs, back pain and sciatica; joint problems, including arthritis; and injuries like sprained ankles, tennis elbow, dislocations and cartilage problems. They also treat strokes, head injuries, multiple sclerosis, fractures, the after-effects of hip-replacement surgery, bronchitis, asthma, pneumonia and cystic fibrosis.

People in middle age and beyond who are so stiff around the neck that, for example, they cannot reverse a car without turning their whole bodies around instead of just their heads often believe themselves victims of irreversible age-related decay. Physiotherapy, however, can often give them fuller, healthier functioning. Physiotherapists also often do preventive work, teaching patients how to avoid a recurrence of damage or injury.

You can find a qualified physiotherapist by contacting the Chartered Society of Physiotherapy★ or the Organisation of Chartered Physiotherapists in Private Practice.★

Some doctors now also do training themselves in such alternative and/or complementary approaches to treatment as acupuncture, autogenic training, biofeedback and clinical hypnosis. Others make available, refer to or recommend approaches ranging from the Alexander Technique to meditation, yoga, ta'i chi, reflexology, therapeutic massage and aromatherapy to help patients recover from illnesses or cope with problems. You will find further details of all the therapies mentioned above (including how to find properly trained practitioners), and of some of the conditions for which they may be particularly helpful, under the heading Therapies and relaxation techniques in the next chapter.

CHAPTER 7

GOOD STRESS GUIDE

STRESS makes the world go round. Without enough of it, we would be disinclined even to get up in the mornings and, when we did, we would find ourselves underperforming for the rest of the day. Yet stress also has a deserved reputation as a destroyer of health and happiness.

If too little stress can give us that can't-be-bothered feeling, and too much is as bad or worse, then the right level for optimum health and performance must lie somewhere between. The perfect balance varies widely from person to person. Some of us thrive in overdrive, while others just find themselves longing for the merry-go-round to stop. Most of us find our ideal levels change from one type of stress to another. Some people who perform brilliantly at work when everything is chaos and crisis, for example, may crumble at home under the stress of the slightest domestic disagreement; or vice versa.

We live in an age where the pace of life seems to be accelerating all the time and when competitiveness and the need to succeed are widely valued. These conditions often lead to inappropriate levels of stress – and that is a risk factor for coronary heart disease, high blood pressure, stroke, diabetes, peptic ulcers, asthma and atherosclerosis. Some medical authorities believe stress is a factor in cancer, and most hold that it depresses the performance of the immune system, making us prone to infection, particularly from viruses.

Women under stress may suffer from menstrual disorders, premenstrual syndrome, pelvic pain and failure to ovulate. Men may have stress-related impotence problems. Men and women may find stress depresses libido and gives them skin and sleep

THE STRESS EFFICIENCY CURVE

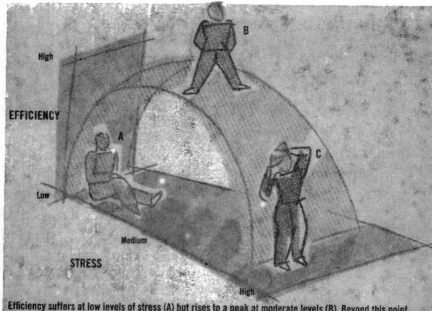

Efficiency suffers at low levels of stress (A) but rises to a peak at moderate levels (B). Beyond this point further arousal results in confusion, and efficiency falls off again (C).

disorders, indigestion, headaches, cramps, back and neck pain, upset stomachs, irritable bowel syndrome, nausea, heartburn, diarrhoea, constipation or flatulence.

In a survey done by the mental-health charity MIND* published in 1992, one-fifth of companies blamed stress-related illness for up to 50 per cent of days that employees took off as sick days. Some estimates have put the percentage of the illnesses reported to GPs which are stress-related as high as 75 per cent.

What is stress?

Stress might have had a long reign as a buzz word in medical, media, psychological and business circles, but it is still imperfectly understood. One of the pioneers of the study of stress, Dr Hans Selye, defined it as 'the rate of wear and tear on the body'. Many contemporary researchers would be more inclined to extend that definition to 'the rate of wear and tear on body and mind'.

We still know more about what it does than we do about exactly how it does it. But the story goes something like this.

Our survival as a species owes much to the fight-or-flight response with which our cave-dwelling forebears generally responded to the novel, the unexpected and the potentially threatening. In evolutionary terms, we are just an eyeblink down the line, still tending to respond to a deadline at work or to worry about how to keep up the mortgage payments with the same action-readying surge of chemicals with which primitive man responded to threat. We respond to emotional stress as if it were physical danger.

There are problems with this. The fight-or-flight response readies us for intense short-term action. We still turn it on to deal with long-term inaction. Our ancestor with the tiger in the corner of his cave had a physical outlet to burn up the extra energy his body produced to ready him for flight: he ran. We are left with a chemical surge raging round our bodies and no automatic way to work off its effects.

When our brains perceive that a demand or a threat is one we can't cope with without going into overdrive, we automatically flip the switch that turns on the stress response. The message goes in the form of small electrical impulses from brain to body organs. When the impulses arrive at the end points of their journeys, small amounts of chemical neurotransmitters are released onto the cells of target organs, which as a result change their mode of functioning.

A back-up message circulates through the body in the form of a hormone (or chemical messenger) released from endocrine glands and circulated through the body via the blood supply to reinforce these changes and add a few of its own. Some of the changes resulting from the electrical messages are often abrupt muscle contractions and high muscle activity enabling us to react quickly to further stimuli. Blood pressure rises, sometimes to quite high levels. It may remain high for some time, and that may damage our arteries.

The heart rate also tends to change. We are often aware that our hearts seem to race after a shock, or to slow right down and beat forcefully if we think that something we fear is about to happen. To ready us for yet more muscle action, blood is diverted from skin and gut to the muscle of the trunk and limbs. This involves blood vessels in the muscles opening up to allow the increased flow, while those in the abdomen and skin contract to divert the flow.

Sweating increases in areas such as the skin around the mouth and nose, the temples, the armpits and between the legs. The palms of the hands and soles of the feet are particularly prone to feeling damp. Saliva, on the other hand, dries up. Gastric acid secretion increases and the stomach may become flabby; we may actually get a sinking feeling in the stomach. Meanwhile, the intestines become more active and we may be aware of them churning and gurgling. Fright can cause an urge to open the bowels, and if the fright is severe enough we may actually lose control. The same goes for the bladder.

Even the sensory organs become involved. The pupils of the eye, for example, dilate to let in more light. The stress hormones, the most important of which in humans is adrenaline, act a little less immediately because blood circulation is a slower messenger system than transmission of nerve impulses. Generally, however, they reinforce and augment the initial response and expand the bronchi (breathing tubes) to allow more air to be taken into the lungs. Adrenaline also affects the metabolic balance of the body, mobilising reserves of energy in the liver and muscles, making glucose available for immediate energy needs.

We all have our own distinctive patterns of these possible responses to stress. Some of us, for example, sweat little but find our pulses race. Others react the other way around. We also vary in the extent to which we become habituated or adapted to repetition of the same stress stimuli. Some of us − consciously or unconsciously − learn more quickly than others when a perceived threat does not materialise that we do not need to continue to react to it each time we encounter it. This has important implications for the way we learn to manage stress successfully. Lack of adaptation may mean we continue to respond to stimuli which are not threatening with an inappropriate stress response quite unnecessarily and damagingly.

Habituation nonetheless may be able to be learned consciously. Laboratory studies have found, for example, that people who

THE STRESS RESPONSE

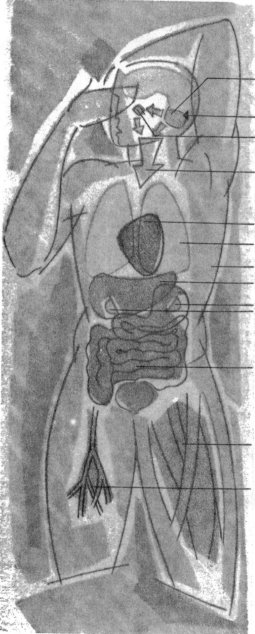

Hypothalamus.

Source of stress response.

Pituitary.

Triggering of
stress response
via nervous system and
hormones.

Heart beats faster. Blood
pressure increases.
Breathing becomes faster
and shallower.

Sweating.

Liver releases energy
stores into blood.

Adrenal glands release
stress hormones such as
adrenaline and
noradrenaline.

Blood is diverted from
the gut to the muscles.

Muscles become tense;
their blood and oxygen
supply is increased.

Blood clots more easily.
Fats and sugars released
into the blood as sources
of energy.

practise meditation or relaxation are better able to adapt to noise stimuli. This may be important for people who live in noisy places, such as near airports or busy roads, and find the noise distressing. It may also have wider implications for learning to deal with other types of stress.

We know, too, that habituation can be suddenly reversed when something happens to give a situation a changed significance for us. For example, someone living near a motorway may manage to become quite desensitised to noise from it but find that seeing or even learning of a bad crash there reactivates a stressful level of awareness of the noise.

Other variables influence our responses to sources of stress. The first time we experience something is likely to be the worst, since we don't know quite what to expect and therefore what strategy will be appropriate for dealing with it. As well as novelty, our perception of stress depends on how important we feel the situation is for us. It is more stressful, for example, to be held up in traffic if it threatens to make us late for an interview for a job we desperately want than if we are being delayed on the way to a meeting we didn't want to go to in the first place.

The level of stress tends to correlate with the duration. We may daydream away the first few minutes stuck in a traffic jam, but feel the tension building up to blow-up level if it goes on for half an hour. Frequency, too, can be a factor. Even short delays in traffic can become stressful if one ends just for the next to begin. Uncertainty can magnify the stress response. If we don't know whether we are going to be held up for three minutes or thirty, we may react initially just as strongly, regardless of the eventual outcome.

Recognising stress

Here are some of the symptoms that might help you to recognise whether you are suffering from levels of stress that are inappropriate for you:

- tightness, discomfort, or even pain in the chest
- rapid or pounding heartbeat
- fainting, or feeling faint

- difficulty sleeping or sleeping too much
- stomach upsets
- indigestion
- nausea
- dry mouth
- a choking feeling
- sweaty palms
- lack of energy
- clenched jaws
- grinding teeth
- tremors and twitches
- headaches
- muscle aches and tension
- frequent urination
- breathlessness or hyperventilation (breathing too quickly and shallowly)
- a niggling accumulation of small discomforts and complaints
- loss of appetite or overeating
- drinking and/or smoking too much
- nervousness
- anxiety
- feeling down in the dumps
- mood swings
- irritability
- difficulty concentrating
- outbursts of anger for no real reason.

The relationship between stress and all its symptoms can be complex and interactional. Disturbed sleep, for example, can be caused by stress and can in itself be stressful. Going to work after a broken night's sleep, perhaps caused by a bad day at work the previous day, can make us more susceptible to being easily upset by anything that goes wrong at work the morning after.

Perhaps the relationship is at its most circular in the area of pain. Stress can cause pain. Suffering pain is stressful, and worrying about what the pain is signalling can add more stress. But being physically tense for long enough can cause aches and pains, or make existing pain worse. Studies have found that if people with chronic pain learn relaxation techniques, they can reduce the severity with which they themselves rate their pain by between 15 per cent and 25 per cent immediately. On the other hand, worrying about what is causing pain or how long it will last or if it is curable, or feeling stressed for other reasons unrelated to the pain itself, can all make it much worse.

Sources of stress

Life events

Dr Thomas Holes and Dr Richard Rahe did research in the US in the late 1960s into the life events most likely to induce stress and how each of them rated. As a result of their work, they published a 'social readjustment rating scale' in the *Journal of Psychosomatic Research* which continues to be a valuable ready reckoner of stress risk (see Table 1, opposite).

Some sources of stress are obvious, such as death, divorce, imprisonment, injury or job loss. Others are less so. Even the anticipation and events connected with Christmas and going on holiday add some points to your stress-risk rating. Change does not have to be for the worse to make a contribution to how stressed we are. Marrying, however happily, is rated enough of an upheaval to add 50 points as reckoned in the rating scale – half the number for death of a spouse.

The point of the scale is to calculate how much at risk you are of developing stress-related illness as a result of what has happened in your life in the past year. It is not making predictions about what will inevitably happen, just warning what the probability is. Individuals vary, anyway, in their natural resilience to a battering by the fates.

If the scale suggests you are at high risk, and you respond by taking extra steps to take care of yourself – by deciding to make changes in your life, by a conscientious programme of relaxation techniques, perhaps by seeking the help of a counsellor or therapist to see you through the rough patch – you can tip the odds back more in your favour.

So using the scale can provide a useful early-warning system. Just tick off which of the events in the chart have happened to you in the past year and add up the points alongside them.

Table 1: STRESS-RATING SCALE

Events	Stress points
Death of spouse	100
Divorce	73
Marital separation	65
Jail term	63
Death of close family member	63
Personal injury or illness	53
Marriage	50
Loss of job	47
Marital reconciliation	45
Retirement	45
Change in health of family member	44
Pregnancy	39
Sexual difficulties	39
Gain of new family member	39
Business readjustment	39
Change of financial state	38
Death of close friend	37
Change in number of arguments with spouse	35
Large mortgage	31
Foreclosure of mortgage or loan	30
Change in responsibilities at work	29
Son or daughter leaving home	29
Trouble with in-laws	28
Outstanding personal achievement	28
Wife begins or stops work	26
Begin or end of school	26
Change of living conditions	25
Revision of personal habits	24
Trouble with boss	23
Change in work hours or conditions	20
Change in residence	20
Change in schools	20
Change in recreation	19
Change in church/social activities	19
Low mortgage or loan	18
Change in sleeping habits	17
Change in number of family gatherings	16
Change in eating habits	15
Vacation	13
Christmas	12
Minor violations of the law	11

This is what your results mean:

- **Fewer than 150:** You have an average chance of developing a stress-related illness.
- **Between 150 and 299:** You are at moderate risk.
- **300 or more:** You are at higher-than-average risk of developing a stress-related illness in the coming months.

Life style

An unhealthy life style is inherently more stressful than a healthy one. In addition, it depresses one's ability to cope with other sources of stress.

A poor diet, smoking (including passively), too much caffeine and alcohol, and a lack of regular exercise all make our lives more stressful and make us less able to cope with stress from other sources. Some people react to stress by drinking too heavily – thereby adding yet another source of stress not only to their own lives but also to the lives of those closest to them. (Chapter 4 says more about sensible alcohol limits and where to turn for help if you find you are exceeding them and cannot stop, or if your partner or someone in your family has a drink problem.)

How much support we have around us – from the nuclear family, through the extended family and into the wider community – and how able we are to draw on what is available also affect the level of stress in our lives.

A study published in the late 1970s found that unemployed people who lacked social support from family, friends and the community had significantly poorer emotional and physical health on a number of measures, including incidence of depression, number of illnesses reported and perception of financial deprivation. A follow-up study of survivors of Norwegian prisoners of war in Nazi concentration camps published a few years earlier found that those who managed to maintain close ties with family, friends or religious or political groups were more likely to survive and better able to adjust to normal life on release.

Money worries are often a major stress factor for people who are out of work. But concern about having enough money to keep up with current spending can be a source of stress for people with jobs, too. Having been caught in a no-win situation, such as being lumbered with a large mortgage on a house after its value has dropped dramatically below the buying price, for example, is more likely to be stressful than a mortgage the same size without the added burden of negative equity.

Life stage

Potential sources of stress change from decade to decade throughout our lives. Caring for young children may be physically demanding, but many families find the psychological drain on their energies increases when youngsters become teenagers – only to be surprised by how much they actually miss loud music, slammed doors and emotional fireworks when those teenagers grow into adults and leave home.

Empty-nest syndrome is, however, by no means universal. Some parents find themselves wishing grown-up sons and daughters would get jobs, pack their bags and set up homes of their own. Couples who suddenly have no one around but one another may enter a new, rich stage in their relationship – or find themselves unable to postpone any longer facing the fact that their emotional cupboard is actually rather bare.

A longed-for 'second honeymoon' might fail to materialise when elderly parents need care just as grown-up children are able to launch out and run their own lives. Women looking forward to a second crack at a career after motherhood may be particularly disappointed to find themselves becoming carers for elderly family members instead. And if they refuse to take on that role, even if they feel certain they have done the reasonable and sensible thing under the circumstances, they may still suffer stressful guilt.

Becoming in-laws can be stressful, too. Tensions may well crop up in families over children's choices of partners and in building the new relationships they entail. Even when parents think their children have made inspired matches with wonderful partners, there is still a chain reaction of readjustments of relationships to accommodate the new unit inside the wider family. With all the goodwill in the world, it can be a bumpy ride.

Not everyone initially takes becoming a grandparent in his or her stride, either. While many men and women are absolutely delighted, for others it feels like being pitched prematurely into an alien age group. Although some grandparents long to see more of their grandchildren than they do, even quite doting ones may have the opposite problem. For them, negotiating just how available they are prepared to be as baby-sitters can be something of a minefield.

The implications of being single can change with the passing decades, too. People who experience the lack of ties through their 20s and 30s as a pleasurable freedom may find it transmuted into yearning for a family life and even into fear of a lonely old age by the time they reach their 40s or 50s or beyond. With marriage break-up becoming so much a feature of life in the 1990s, increasing numbers of people are finding themselves single again after decades of marriage, and not necessarily through choice. That can mean starting over, to build a new life to replace the old.

Women who breezed through their 20s and 30s defining themselves as child-free may begin to redefine themselves as childless as 40 approaches and they sense the biological clock ticking away their last fertile years. They may begin to worry about not having children, and agonise over whether to try to grab this last chance. (See Chapter 5 for more about the pros and cons of deciding to have a baby at 40-plus.)

For some people, the middle years of their lives can be a time of agonising over how far short of their early plans and expectations their lives and careers have fallen and how little time they may have left. What, they ask themselves, has happened to those early dreams of living happily-ever-after? Why haven't they reached the top of the professional ladder? Made the scientific breakthrough of their generation? Written the novel of the decade?

For others, it can be a time when achievement has peaked and the worry is how to continue to sit on top of what feels like an increasingly greasy pole as younger rivals climb up and make (or are perceived to be making) assaults on it. Worse, it can be a time of having no job at all and wondering whether you will ever again.

Retirement, too, means different things to different people. It can be something planned for and looked forward to for years before. Or it can be an unwelcome decline in an ex-worker's quality of life. Probably the most stressful scenario is when retirement comes out of the blue, earlier than expected and with no time to plan or adjust to the idea.

Some people fear ageing, which they see as losing looks, health, strength, potency, power, competitive edge, promotion prospects or just running out of time. Deaths of parents, friends or contemporaries can leave us grieving not only for our loss but, increasingly, also for our own mortality.

The environment

Our physical environment can be a plus or a minus for stress. A noisy road or air traffic or neighbours, overcrowded conditions, damp homes, a long and difficult journey to and from work and a polluted urban atmosphere are just some of the sources of environmental stress.

Interestingly, however, too little happening around us is no better than too much. Clinical studies have shown that, deprived of sufficient stimulation, we react (in extreme cases) to the sensory deprivation by becoming bored and finally by hallucinating. If too little is demanded of our minds, they invent processing tasks by imagining stimuli that don't actually exist in order to give themselves some work to do.

The social environment, too, can contribute to stress. Not getting on with the neighbours can be stressful; discord with people within the same household can be even more so. People confronting racial discrimination and even harassment on a daily basis are living extremely stressful lives. So are those who are afraid to go out because they fear becoming victims of crime.

The individual

Stress is, to some extent, all in the mind. How much stress we experience is more closely related to the way we perceive and respond to what is going on in our lives than it is to the objective facts of what is actually happening to us. The way we perceive is, in turn, a product of a number of different factors, including our memories, the way we anticipate the future, and our habitual ways of thinking and reacting. To some extent, how stressed we feel depends on the way we think about things.

Research into individual responses to stress has been heavily influenced by the work of two American researchers, Dr Meyer Friedman and Dr Ray Rosenman, who investigated the link between personality type and the likelihood of a heart attack. They published the results of their research, which was on men only, in the *Journal of the American Medical Association* in 1959. They found that what they called Type A people were three times as likely as Type B people to have heart attacks. But they also found that if Type A people deliberately modified their behaviour to be more like that of Type Bs, the Type As reduced their heart-attack risk.

According to the study, Type A people were very competitive, strong, forceful personalities who did everything, including speaking, quickly, and were strivers for promotion at work, social advancement and public recognition. They were restless when not active, seemed to thrive on doing more than one thing at a time, were punctual, enjoyed meeting deadlines and were impatient with delays and were easily angered.

Type Bs, on the other hand, were easy-going or retiring, methodical, content with their status, were slow to anger, enjoyed doing nothing, were happiest doing one thing at a time, didn't rush, were patient and not easily upset, were often late and inclined to disregard time and ignore deadlines, and were not competitive at sports or at work.

Most people, however, don't fit neatly into one category or the other. You probably thought as you read the above that you seemed something of a mixture yourself, although possibly you recognised one or the other style as predominating. Subsequent studies this side of the Atlantic have failed to find the categories particularly relevant to heart disease patterns in the UK or elsewhere in Europe. The persistence of the Type A versus Type B model's influence on thinking about stress stems not so much from the research results it has generated here as from the fact that it is a nice, neat model and easy to teach to medical students, for whom it remains on the curriculum.

Despite the hold that the Type A versus Type B paradigm still seems to have on thinking about how stress arises from individual differences, a more subtle and useful approach to understanding how we contribute to our own experience of stress may come from looking at the highly individual ways in which we interpret what is happening to us. The extent to which altering the way we think and act can change the way we feel, and how that can lead to better strategies for coping with stress, is discussed in the Stress-watch section, below.

The workplace

Some jobs are intrinsically stressful. Among the worst are air traffic control, flying aircraft, police work, mining, advertising, acting, dentistry and journalism. Many managers in the increasingly competitive world of business, too, suffer considerable stress. This is particularly true of those who have to spend large chunks of their lives in airports, aircraft and hotels.

Not having enough to do at work, or finding what you have to do is not challenging enough, is stressful. So is working long hours spent trying to keep up with an unrealistic workload. However, workaholism can sometimes be less a product of the workplace than a symptom of not coping in other areas of one's life. The workaholic may be taking refuge from difficulties outside work by becoming overabsorbed in the job.

Changes in technology can be stressful, as can unpleasant physical surroundings, whether they are dingy and cramped or too bright and noisy. Shift work imposes particular pressures of its own because it disrupts the body's natural rhythms, in much the same way as jet lag does, adding physical sources of stress to potential psychological ones. People do seem to adapt reasonably well eventually if they are on a fixed-shift pattern, but not if they are on rotating shifts.

Uncertainty is a major contributor to stress at work. People who are unclear about what is expected of them or what the purpose of their job really is, those who are unable to contribute to workplace decisions, and those left in the dark or in confusion by ineffective internal communications are all more vulnerable to stress. So are people who fail to be given an expected promotion, or see little prospects of career development ahead of them.

There can be extra stresses for women, especially if they work in fields traditionally seen as men's work or move into more senior positions where they have men working (sometimes reluctantly) for them. They may suffer or feel they are suffering from discrimination on sex grounds when they try to rise higher in the organisation and hit the 'glass ceiling', or are subjected to sexual harassment.

Conflicts between the demands of family and job are also a regular source of frustration which particularly affects women. Many women live on a tightrope, balancing feelings of guilt that they are not putting more of their time into mothering against worries that family demands prevent them being totally committed to their jobs. These feelings of guilt may persist even when women are giving every bit as much of themselves to their jobs as male colleagues are.

What sometimes results is the 'superwoman syndrome', when working women attempt to prove to themselves and the world that they can have brilliant careers while being wonderful wives, perfect mothers, immaculate housekeepers and inspired hostesses. For such women, even trivial domestic tasks can end up with higher priority than their own physical and psychological well-being. It is potentially a recipe for eventual crack-up.

Stresswatch

Keeping stress at a healthy level involves knowing when there is too much or too little in your life – see the list of possible symptoms above – and being clued up about what you can do to reduce or increase it. Finally, you need to know your way around the various techniques for coping with unavoidable stress.

Understress
If your problem is that you are not under enough stress (because life seems to lack challenge or significant interest, or just to be making too few demands on you), you might want to look at your life style and at yourself to see what changes you might want to make. The aim of the exercise is to be less comfortable and secure than you are, and there can be many routes to achieving this. What can you do to change your routine and bump yourself out of that comfortable rut? What can you try that is new for you and interesting, challenging, even risky?

Some possibilities might be changing your job to something more demanding, applying for promotion where you are, finding out about training or adult education courses that might make you eligible for a step up the ladder at work, or taking up a new interest. Additionally, you might want to do a course in something just because it interests you, or to take on something voluntary.

Is there something you have always really wanted to do but

found endless reasons not to start yet? Now could be the time. (Chapter 8 will give you more ideas to consider.)

Overstress

If you feel you have too much stress in your life at the moment, this section is for you. After you have examined the sources of stress in your life, the next step is to see which ones you can eliminate or better control. Then you can turn your attention to learning how to cope better with what's left.

Most life events, such as death and illness, don't give us a great deal of choice. The life stage we are in is open to negotiation only up to a point, although there are some possibilities for action here. For example, pre-retirement courses, where they are available and circumstances permit them, can minimise the stress of the transition from working to post-working life.

The way we think about what is happening can determine how stressful it is, even if we can do nothing to change it. We can, for example, worry just as much about adult children as we did when they were younger. But if we can accept that however much we worry we aren't responsible for them, it can take some of the stress out of watching them make different choices from the ones we wish they would make.

Whatever stage we are at in our lives, a corrosive source of stress that often goes unacknowledged is not knowing where we want to go from here. If this applies to you, there is a section on goal planning in the next chapter you might find useful.

Life style is one of the stress sources that most lends itself to voluntary change. We can decide whether to exercise regularly, eat healthily, drink moderately, give up smoking if we haven't yet and avoid passive smoking if we have, and generally take better care of ourselves. We can be more aware of the potential resource of the help and support of family and friends, and make use of it when we need to. A problem shared can be a problem robbed of its ability to generate stress by circling in an endless loop in our heads.

If a financial muddle causes stress, facing up to the facts and planning the way forward – however painful – with the help, if needed, of a debt counsellor (via Citizens Advice Bureaux*) can come as a great relief.

One individual source of potential stress lies in our perception of what is happening to us. It is what we think about what is happening, rather than what is actually happening, that influences how we feel about it. This apparently simple yet subtle insight underlies cognitive therapy, rated by a number of studies as the psychological treatment of choice for depression and one increasingly widely used for other behavioral and mood disorders.

The underlying principle is equally applicable to stress. For example, in a new, challenging situation there are any number of possible internal dialogues we might have going on in our heads. Among them could be: 'I know I cannot cope with this. I am going to be a complete failure'; or: 'This is difficult. All I can do is try the best I can'; or: 'Isn't this exciting, having the chance to try to do this? I might really learn something from it.'

Each of these responses will produce a different level of internal stress, not to mention a different likelihood of success or failure, with the further stress implications that has. An excellent book, *Feeling Good – The New Mood Therapy**, by David D. Burns, is aimed specifically at self-treating depression. But many of the principles outlined in it and the exercises given could easily be adapted to dealing with an excess of stress, even when stress is not manifesting itself, as it sometimes does, as depression. Another extremely helpful book by Burns, *The Feeling Good Handbook**, gives self-help suggestions and exercises for learning to deal with stress and anxiety arising from a number of different sources, including fear of public speaking and interviews, procrastination and lack of self-esteem.

The stress that comes from fear of crime can be minimised in two ways. The first is to understand more about what the danger actually is. The second is to take steps to be better able to defend yourself. Many people, as they grow older, increasingly fear that they are likely to become victims of house or street crime. The truth is that, even after allowing for the fact that some older people are staying at home out of fear, people between 16 and 30 are six times more at risk of becoming a victim of crime than those who are over 60.

Nevertheless, being a victim of crime – at any age – is extremely stressful. The voluntary agency Victim Support* can help if it happens to you. Advice about door and window locks, chains, peepholes and so on to make houses more secure is available free from police Crime Prevention Officers all over the country. In many parts of the country, self-defence classes are available. The local police or local library may have details of them.

Self-defence

There are a few simple measures you can take to make yourself less vulnerable – and so less anxious – when you are out. They include:

- Park your car in a well-lit area when you can.
- Reverse in if you are leaving your car in a car park. Then if when you return to collect your car you are, for example, uncomfortable about someone loitering nearby, you can get away quickly.
- Approach your parked car with your keys already in your hand for the same reason.
- Always lock yourself in the car. Get into the habit of doing it even before you belt up or turn the key in the ignition.
- Never leave anything tempting visible in the car whether you are in it or leaving it. When you are driving, a handbag is less of a temptation on the floor than on the passenger seat.
- Walk on the lit side of the road if possible, and keep away from hedges or walls you cannot see behind.
- Carry a personal alarm if you feel nervous about where you are going.

Stress at work

Reducing stress at work might involve being prepared to have a hard and honest look at what role we want work to have in our lives and measuring it against the one it has now, and, if necessary, making changes.

If you are finding work stressful because you don't understand exactly what is expected of you, ask. If you would like training and the chance to do something more challenging, say so. Seek advice about what sort of training you could arrange for yourself that would improve your promotion prospects. If your firm has an appraisal scheme, you might ask if you could have your next one now instead of having to wait until it is due.

If you can't ask, consider doing some assertiveness training; you will find this equally useful in personal relationships. (An excellent do-it-yourself book on the subject is *A Woman in Your Own Right*** by Anne Dickson. Men would find the techniques outlined in the book useful, too.)

Try to listen to what you say to yourself when you are criticised at work. If your boss says he or she is unhappy with a report you have written, do you hear that s/he is unhappy with the report or that you are a failure? Do you say to yourself that you have written a report that is not up to scratch, or that you are stupid and can never do anything right? Do you feel that nothing you do ever pleases your boss, or that you might be able to learn something about how to do better reports from what s/he has to say?

If, after hearing what your boss has to say, you honestly still think the report is a good one, say so. If you can't, re-read the remarks about assertiveness above.

Do you believe that you must do everything perfectly every time? It is good to have high standards, but it is a stress time-bomb to think you are never allowed to make a mistake. Discover how, when you do make a mistake, you can see it as a chance for learning, rather than as a personal failure. Learn to see a crisis at work as an opportunity rather than a disaster: it is a chance to do things differently from the way they have always been done before. Brilliant careers have risen out of the ashes of such apparent low points.

When there are situations you are unhappy about at work but really can do nothing to change, the healthy low-stress response is to accept that you cannot do anything and let go worrying. You may know that, but ask yourself if you are really doing it.

Managing time

Good time management can remove much of the stress from work. It can mean getting more done in a day. It can even mean working so much more efficiently that you shorten an overlong working day, thus reducing another source of stress. Management of your private time can also help to fit the various components of your life together in a way that minimises the total amount of stress.

Start every day with a list of things you would like to do that day. Is it realistic? If it isn't, decide what matters least and delete it. Arrange what's left by coding with a colour, a number or an initial what is urgent but unimportant, urgent and important, important but not urgent, and neither important nor urgent, and then decide in what order it makes sense to tackle them.

Make sure you give priority to at least some important but not urgent items as well as urgent ones, especially the ones that involve forward planning. Tick items off as you do them. That way, if you don't get everything done, you will ensure that what is carried over is what mattered the least to do that day, and you won't always be pushing important work to the bottom of the pile. You can review relative importance and urgency again at the beginning of the next day.

If you feel you are just not getting through enough in a day, have another look at whether what you are trying to do is unrealistic. If it isn't, have a look at the list of top time-wasters below and see which ones apply to you:

- interruptions, including the telephone
- indecision
- overlong or unnecessary meetings
- not having a plan for the day
- not having an organised desk or work area
- not being able to say 'no'
- not being able to ask for or accept help
- flitting from job to job without finishing anything
- not being able to find people when you need to
- chatting too much
- poor communications at home or at work
- jumping into tasks without planning them
- indulging in 'if onlys' – in time spent thinking how different things would be if only ...

When you have worked out which of the above are wasting most of your time, you can start doing something about them. Which ones are unavoidable and which can you change? For example, if the telephone constantly interrupts you at work, is it essential that you answer it all the time? Or could you arrange a period in the day when you don't and use it to tackle demanding jobs for which you really need an uninterrupted stretch of time.

Perhaps the most effective way to find out which of the time-wasters apply to you may be to keep a time log for a couple of weeks first. If you have never done this before, you may be amazed to discover where your time really goes. All you need is a chart like the one below. If you are using it outside working hours, or to cover both working and non-working time, you might need to extend the times it covers accordingly.

To use the log:

- List anything that takes five minutes or more as a major activity.
- Code interruptions to working time – for example, with a P for something personal and a T for a telephone call.
- Note approximate duration beside each major activity and each interruption.
- Once an interruption runs for more than five minutes, indicate with an arrow over to the adjacent column that it has become a major activity.

Once you have collected the data for two weeks, you can set about finding where your time really goes and how you can use it better. You can look at why you do things the way you do – because you are in the habit of doing them that way or because it is an efficient way to do them – and see how you might do them better. You may see that it makes sense to do chores in a different order, or that it would be more efficient to group some tasks together.

TIME LOG

Date:_____

Time	Major activities	Interruptions
8.30		
9.30		
10.30		
11.30		
12.30		
1.30		
2.30		
3.30		
4.30		
5.30		

It can improve your efficiency enormously if (at work and outside working hours) you do the exercise and then repeat it about once a year, to check if you are falling back into old bad habits or have invented any new ones.

Coping with stress

Once you have explored sources of overstress in your life and thought about what changes you may be able to make to minimise them, you may well find yourself still left with a level of stress that is too high for comfort. There may be nothing for it but to learn to live with, at least from time to time, more stress than you would wish. The following sections will help you limit the damage to health and happiness.

Taking time out

If stress is beginning to get on top of you, stop for a few minutes. A few slow, deep breaths and a stepping back from what you are doing, figuratively at least, can help get priorities into perspective before you plunge back into the fray again.

Breathing is a key technique in dealing on the spot with any situation that arouses anxiety, as well as being good longer-term therapy for on-going stress. What most of us do when something frightens or worries us is make it 10 times worse by immediately going into a pattern of hyperventilating – breathing shallowly and fast. The antidote is to breathe very slowly and deliberately, taking the air down so deeply that if we put our hands on our ribs at about waist level we feel the ribs pushing the hands out as we breathe in.

The best way to be able to use this technique when we need it is to practise at times when we feel quite relaxed and unthreatened until it becomes quite automatic. Then we can switch into the mode at will, even when we feel anxious. It is best to practise for a few minutes at a time standing, with hands on the ribs to check they are expanding as they should. Breathe in for a count of three or four, and out for the same again. When you have mastered that (and as long as you do not have any breathing problems such as asthma), you might want to increase the number of counts in stages up to about seven.

When we become anxious in a crisis, we cannot really start thinking clearly about the best way to handle things until after we have managed to use our breathing to calm us down. For a full-blown panic attack, the same deep, slow breathing is helpful, as long as we have practised it enough beforehand to be able to turn it on even under major stress.

Breathing into and from a paper bag (held over nose and mouth) for about a minute can be remarkably effective first aid. Some people prone to panic attacks find carrying a paper bag in a pocket or handbag enables them to treat themselves instantly if they have an attack; it also may make them feel more secure just knowing it is there. It is a useful option for people who panic only in limited and quite specific situations, for example as part of a strategy for conquering fear of flying.

A good night's sleep is also an excellent antidote to stress, but it can be an early casualty when stress sets in.

Dealing with sleep problems

Stress can cause sleep problems and sleep problems increase stress. Here are some tips that can help break that vicious circle:

- Try to have a routine and stick to it. Ideally it should include going to bed and getting up at the same time every day and a ban on daytime naps.
- Check your bed and bedding. Are they comfortable enough?
- Is your bedroom a comfortable temperature?
- Try a milky bedtime drink.
- Keep off coffee, and ideally tea as well, after about mid-afternoon.
- Eat light and early in the evenings.
- Exercise helps, whether you take it in the evening or even early in the day.
- If you find cleaning your teeth or showering at bedtime wakes you up, do it earlier.
- Try a soak in a hot bath last thing at night.
- Keep entertainment that is stressful or exciting out of the bedroom. Don't watch or listen to the news last thing. Stick to light, undemanding (even boring) reading and/or a relaxation technique (see below).

- Clear the mental decks as much as you can before you go to bed. If you are worried about how many things you have to do next day, write a list.
- Keep a pad and pen by your bed. If ideas or things you have to remember next day pop into your head, write them down.
- If you can't get off to sleep, get up. Make a warm drink. Perhaps read for a while. Wait until you feel sleepy before trying again.
- Remember that most people who have trouble sleeping actually sleep more than they think. Even when they are certain they have not closed their eyes all night, they almost certainly have slept, and probably for some hours.

Deep breathing is good first aid for stress and sleep is a good preventative measure and remedy. Stress-proofing our lives can also include using one of a number of relaxation techniques on a regular basis and, if needed, seeking outside help.

Below are some possibilities.

Therapies and relaxation techniques

If you found that you had symptoms listed in the section Recognising stress, above, it may be advisable to talk to your GP about them. This is especially important if your symptoms included the first one in the list – tightness, discomfort or pains in the chest.

Unfortunately, the only help many doctors offer patients for stress itself is tranquillisers (such as diazepam and lorazepam) for the symptoms of stress and anxiety. They can help as first aid to get you through a crisis, but will do nothing to help you sort out underlying causes. And they are addictive. If your doctor prescribes them, they should be a low dose and for days only.

Some GP practices now offer counselling or psychotherapy, which can help patients explore underlying causes of stress and look at how they can change what they can and cope with what they cannot. But such practices are still in a minority. Some may offer acupuncture or hypnosis or massage, but, again, this is not usual. The odds are that if you want to turn to other therapies, you will have to find them and pay for them yourself.

There are a number of possibilities, some of which are listed alphabetically below. They include self-help such as deep relaxation and therapies for mind, body and a combination of the two. Some will help you address causes, others will focus more on effects. Some offer a mixture of the two.

As yet, little regulation of alternative and complementary therapies exists, so training standards vary. However, a number of self-appointed regulating bodies (detailed in the relevant entries below) do cover different therapies and can refer you to practitioners who should have acceptable standards of training. They can also give you an idea of what you can expect to pay. Costs vary not only from therapy to therapy but also from practitioner to practitioner, often depending on where in the country they operate.

Acupuncture

Acupuncture goes back at least as far as 2697 BC, when Huan Ti became emperor of China and, with a contemporary physician, worked out the principles on which the technique is based. Its underlying philosophy is that it harmonises the vital force or energy of the body called chi, which runs along invisible lines called meridians within the healthy body. When chi is not flowing freely, mental or physical illness results.

Acupuncture uses the insertion of needles, or application of heat or fingertip pressure (acupressure), or a combination of all these methods, sometimes along with more modern additions such as the use of electromagnetic fields, polarised light or low-power lasers.

Although seventeenth-century missionaries to China brought word of acupuncture back to Europe, it was not until about 30 to 40 years ago that it really began to catch on with Europeans who were not of Chinese origin. It has been given some credence by Western scientists who have found that the 1000 traditional acupuncture points and 59 meridians of the body do have identifiable electrical properties.

Acupuncture is offered for a wide range of ailments, including stress-related indigestion, anxiety and depression, as well as sprains, fractures (after the bones have set), osteoarthritis, rheumatoid arthritis, headaches, migraine, neuralgia, hiatus hernia, ulcers, bronchitis, asthma, high blood pressure, obesity and various kinds of addictions.

Some GPs are now trained to use acupuncture or make it available at their surgeries, and some NHS hospitals also use it. An alternative is to self-refer to a private practitioner. To find one, contact the Council for Acupuncture★, British Acupuncture Association★ or the Traditional Acupuncture Society★.

Alexander Technique

This technique aims to approach stress symptoms through teaching the correct alignment and use of the body. Last century, an Australian dramatic actor, F.N. Alexander, was trying to work out why he kept losing his voice on stage, and found he had a habit of tossing his head back as he tried to project his voice to the back of the audience. When he corrected his overall posture, without straining or becoming tense, and let his head and neck go into their natural position, not only his voice but also his general health improved. At the turn of the century, he left Australia and began to teach in the UK and the US.

Today, an Alexander Teacher not only takes a case history of past and present problems, but in addition notices posture, signs of stress, voice timbre, mannerisms, gait and overall healthy or otherwise appearance before s/he begins a series of lessons. High blood pressure, spastic colon, asthma, trigeminal neuralgia, osteoarthritis, frequent headaches and lack of energy are all claimed to respond to the Alexander Technique. Find a teacher through the Society of Teachers of the Alexander Technique★.

Aromatherapy

This is massage (see below) using essential oils as well as the stroking and kneading of soft tissues of the body common to other massage techniques. Absorption of the oils through the skin is part of the therapy. Aromatherapy also incorporates some reflexology (see below).

Massage with essential oils is not new. Scent pots were found in Tutankhamen's tomb, and the Greeks and Romans also used oils for massage. A contemporary aromatherapist treating you for stress would take your history, discuss symptoms and any medical problems you have, ascertain any medication you are taking and choose the oil or oils for their relaxing qualities and their appropriateness for you as an individual. He or she will advise you to drink plenty of water (to flush out toxins) but no alcohol (because it could interfere with the therapeutic effects of the oils) for the rest of the day.

To find a qualified aromatherapist, contact the International Federation of Aromatherapists★.

Autogenic training

This method, too, has a good research track record, not only for stress but also for helping overcome or manage various illnesses and psychological problems. It uses phrases such as 'my arm is very warm' and 'my heartbeat is calm and regular' in a series of easy-to-learn mental exercises done for a few minutes at a time several times daily. The exercises are designed to help harmonise mind, body and emotions to reach an altered state of consciousness similar to some meditational states.

There are also what are called 'intentional exercises', which are used to release blocked emotions and are selected as the need arises. Autogenic training's apparent simplicity is deceptive. The technique can be powerful, and it needs a good teacher. Find one who is qualified through the British Association for Autogenic Training and Therapy★.

Biofeedback

This is a way of monitoring training in relaxation by giving feedback on how well we are doing. It can involve devices measuring a number of different responses, including heart rate, blood pressure, muscle tension, electrical activity in the brain, sweating and skin temperature. A lie detector is a biofeedback device that measures the physiology of the stress caused by lying.

Biofeedback therapy has been shown to be useful in conditions like tension headaches, migraine, insomnia, anxiety and high blood pressure, and in combination with other relaxation techniques to reduce the risk of heart attacks. Find out about biofeedback from your GP or from the British Holistic Medical Association★, or the British Complementary Medicine Association★.

A simple and cheap do-it-yourself biofeedback device is a small adhesive patch that measures skin temperature by changing colour. The patches are only an approximate guide. They are also sensitive to ambient temperature, and exercise, drinking and smoking will affect them too. Nevertheless, wearing one can be a useful way to focus on what causes us stress in the course of a day and to get some indication of how successful we are when we are using relaxation techniques. One version is called Biodot and can be obtained from Stresswise★.

Clinical hypnosis

Some doctors and some therapists are trained to use hypnosis as a tool in therapy dealing with stress and other psychosomatic and psychological problems. Learning to hypnotise people is the relatively easy part. The real skill lies in knowing how to use trance, the altered state of awareness that is at once both physically relaxed and mentally alert, and in which the mind is more open to accepting suggestions.

As in the case of psychotherapists generally, training varies widely and there is no legal minimum qualification requirement. So choose your hypnotherapist with care, and don't ask questions just about his or her training in hypnotic techniques, but also about the psychotherapeutic framework within which s/he uses it. Contact the Institute for Complementary Medicine★ and the National Council of Psychotherapists and Hypnotherapy Register★ for more information. (See also Psychotherapy and Self-hypnosis, below.)

Counselling

Counselling can help you to discover the areas in your life that are causing stress and to work out ways of changing or coping with them. Counsellors don't give advice. They are nonjudgmental and respect absolute confidentiality. Many companies now offer free counselling to employees through Employee Assistance Programmes; or you can find a counsellor for yourself through the British Association of Counselling★. If you feel your stress arises from difficulties in your relationship with your partner, you might prefer to try Relate★. Cruse★ specialises in bereavement counselling.

Massage

First accepted by the medical profession as 'scientific' in the last century (it is from massage that the profession of physiotherapy –

see below – evolved), massage is having something of a revival as a therapeutic technique. It is being used for a range of conditions, including asthma, arthritis, rheumatism, backache, headaches, constipation, cramp and insomnia, as well as stress.

It is increasingly being made available on the NHS in hospitals and hospices as well as in doctors' surgeries. Private practitioners can be found at sports centres and beauty clinics, and some do a visiting service to homes and offices. You can even fight stress at work by having someone massage your neck and shoulders while you are sitting at your desk.

One theory about the effectiveness of massage is that it helps to produce endorphins, the brain chemicals that are nature's painkillers. In any case, it is advisable not to eat for a couple of hours before massage or to drink alcohol for the rest of the day. Contact the British Massage Therapy Council* for information about practitioners and organisations.

Meditation

Meditation has scored well in research into the benefits of relaxation techniques. One study found people who meditate use health services 68 per cent less than those who do not. And one Dutch insurance company cut its premiums by 40 per cent for people who meditate.

In meditation, the aim is to reduce the mental 'noise' by focusing the mind on the breath, a mental image such as a flower or a lake, or on a mantra, which can be a sound or a word. When the mind wanders, you gently bring it back to whatever you are focusing on.

Meditation is best learned with the help of a teacher. For information about centres throughout the country, write to Transcendental Meditation*.

Muscle relaxation (active)

Sit or lie somewhere comfortable. If you are lying down, a firm surface is better than one so soft you sink into it deeply. Now, systematically work through the muscles of your legs (feet, ankles, calves, thighs), arms (hands, lower arm, upper arm), trunk and face, first clenching as tight as you can, holding the tension and then releasing. Don't forget shoulders and stomach when you are doing the trunk. They are both places that for many of us hold much of our tension.

Don't rush it. Give yourself at least 20 minutes, longer if you can. (If you suffer from high blood pressure, it is better to avoid tensing and opt for passive relaxation, described below.)

Muscle relaxation (passive)

Sit or lie somewhere comfortable but, again, make sure it is firm. This time, the aim is just to let the tension flow out of muscles one by one all over your body. Again, start with feet, ankles, calves, thighs; move on to hands and arms; then to stomach, back and shoulders; and finally to neck, jaw, mouth, forehead, eyes, cheeks and scalp.

It might help to close your eyes and form a picture of each group of muscles in turn as you are working on them. You might like to visualise them becoming softer and softer. Or as you focus attention on each set in turn, count from one to ten, timing every number to coincide with an exhaled breath, and letting tension go a little more on each count.

Physiotherapy

Physiotherapy is provided at some GP practices and hospitals, where it is less likely to be prescribed for stress itself than for the physical effects of stress, which can include tension, back pain and repetitive strain injury. You can self-refer to physiotherapists in private practice.

Although physiotherapists still use some massage, they also now use manipulation, mobilisation, exercises and sophisticated electrical treatments such as muscle-stimulating currents and ultrasound to promote healing and relieve pain. You can find a qualified physiotherapist by contacting the Chartered Society of Physiotherapy★ or the Organisation of Chartered Physiotherapists in Private Practice★.

Psychotherapy

The most intensive psychotherapy is psychoanalysis, which can involve hour-long sessions four or five times a week over a long period of time. Therapists offering psychoanalysis have been analysed themselves and have had very lengthy training. At the other end of the spectrum are people offering briefer therapy from various theoretical perspectives and with different qualities and quantities of training. Therapists' work can overlap with that of counsellors. Again, what you say will be treated with complete confidentiality.

Some types of psychotherapy have, in common with psycho-analysis, an orientation towards finding causes of present problems in past experience. Others, including cognitive therapy, focus more on how problems are being maintained in the present and on how to make more positive choices in the future.

To find a psychotherapist, contact the UK Council of Psycho-therapists★, the National Council of Psychotherapists★, the British Association for Counselling★ or the Institute for Complementary Medicine★.

Reflexology

This technique is based on the ancient Chinese idea that every part of the body is connected by energy pathways which terminate in the feet, the hands and the head. Thus it is assumed that every part of the body, including the internal organs, is connected with different points on the feet, and that the use of controlled thumb and index finger pressure on the right spot, usually on the feet although it can be on hands or head, can relax tension and stimu-late the health of the corresponding part of the body.

Reflexology is used not only to treat stress but in conjunction with other treatments for headaches, migraine, insomnia, anxiety, depression, backache, stiffness in the neck and shoulders, and other muscular tension. It should not be used for anyone suffering an infectious disease, with a fever or with inflammation of the lymphatic or vein systems, during an unstable pregnancy, or with deep-vein thrombosis or severe cardiac disorder.

Find a qualified reflexologist through the British School of Reflexology★.

Rehearsal

If you have something coming up that you are worried about handling, use visualisation (explained below) to rehearse it, a bit at a time if it lends itself to being divided into stages. First, use deep breathing or muscle relaxation, or visualisation of being somewhere you feel safe and secure, to allow yourself to become relaxed.

It may help to see the coming event as if you were watching yourself on a screen, if you are able. If you find yourself becoming tense, do more relaxation work before you carry on. Don't forget that while you are doing it in your head, you are actor, director and scriptwriter. So make sure you write a successful outcome for yourself and allow a little time to bask in how it feels.

Self-hypnosis

Another good technique for deep relaxation, self-hypnosis can also be used for exploring sources of stress, and is an excellent way to rehearse for potentially stressful events coming up, as described above. There are many books on the subject. One of the best is *Self-Hypnosis, The Complete Manual for Health and Self-change*★★ by Brian M. Altman and Peter T. Lambrou. However, self-hypnosis is best learned from a doctor or psychotherapist trained to use hypnosis therapeutically. (See Clinical hypnosis, above.)

Shiatsu

This ancient Japanese therapy uses oriental massage and finger pressure to stimulate acupuncture points and meridians. It is sometimes described as acupuncture without needles. Over the years it has added aspects of other therapies, including massage. Shiatsu practitioners recommend a natural diet and pay attention to a person's general mental health, as well as using the shiatsu technique. This aims to prevent disease and keep the body in harmony with the environment.

Find a qualified practitioner through the Shiatsu Society★.

T'ai chi

In its present form, t'ai chi dates from 14th-century China, where it was recognised that anxiety and stress, by causing tension, could interfere with healthy body functioning, particularly through its effects on breathing and circulation.

Although t'ai chi looks gentle and easy, it is actually a highly sophisticated system of fluid and shifting movements designed to promote health of mind and body. Unlike in yoga (see below), in t'ai chi the poses are not held and there is no stretching.

You cannot learn t'ai chi from a book, but you can practise it at home once you have learned the 108 basic movements; these are done in one of two possible sequences, one of 100 postures and the other of between 30 and 40. Although it sounds tiring, most people who practise it say they have more energy after a session than before.

T'ai chi imposes no stress on the heart and so is safe for people with heart disorders, hypertension and coronary arterial disease. Find a teacher through the British T'ai Chi Chuan Centre*.

Visualisation

Sit or lie comfortably, close your eyes and imagine, as vividly as you can, being somewhere in which you feel relaxed, comfortable and really safe and secure. It can be somewhere you have only been once, or somewhere you have been often. It can be somewhere you remember from childhood, or somewhere you hope lies in your future. It can be completely a product of your own imagination. It really does not matter which, as long as it has the right associations for you.

Conjure up the sense of being there in as much detail, and involving as many senses, as you can. Try really to visualise it. Become aware of what the surroundings look like, what colours you can see there, what shapes. Then turn your attention to the sounds. If you are out of doors, can you hear the sound of birds? Or if someone is there with you, can you conjure up a voice? How does it feel? Is there a breeze? If there is, can you tell the direction by how it touches your face? And what are the physiological feelings you associate with being in this place? Take time to notice. Are there any tastes you associate with the place or situation? Smells?

It matters less how much you succeed in all these tasks than it does that you become absorbed in attempting them and that you get a sense of being there in whatever way works for you. Most people will find they imagine more vividly in one area of the senses than in the others.

Yoga

Yoga has dual aims. One is to promote physical welfare by exercising the whole body systematically to improve circulation and create a feeling of well-being. In addition, it aims to aid psychological health by sharpening yet calming the mind. As a result, yoga may both reduce stress and help with other ailments.

Again, there are many books and some videos on the subject, but there is no real substitute for going to a teacher, at least to get you started. Most local authorities have classes, or contact the Wheel of Yoga★.

A final warning

Stress is a funny business. The popular misconception that golf is an antidote to stress is disproved by the latest information to come out of Japan, where they are mad about the game. Western golfers may find playing is de-stressing to some extent, because it usually takes their minds off other problems, at least for as long as they are on the course (although playing badly can be stressful in itself). But in Japan golf is intrinsically stressful, even on a good day. Courses are too few, too crowded – and run with military precision. Tee-off times have to be booked as much as six months ahead and are seven minutes apart for the lucky, six for everyone else.

Professional caddies, mostly women, cajole and bully to keep players moving at exactly the right pace to keep their place in the regimented progression around the course. In addition, players tend to smoke, drink and gamble on the outcome. The result is that golf is officially rated six times more likely than running to kill a man over 60 in Japan, and is more apt to be a cause of death than tennis or mountaineering. Recreation doesn't get much more stressful than that!

If you would like to know more about stress, there is also a Which? Consumer Guide called *Understanding Stress*★★.

CHAPTER **8**

LOOKING FORWARD

FOR MOST of us, our future beyond 40 probably depends more on our outlook than on any other single factor. Our health, to some extent, relies on a spin of the roulette wheel. No matter what we do to tilt the odds more in our favour, we may still be unable to protect ourselves against serious illness. Yet, it remains true that, for most of us, it is our outlook that is the largest single influence on how successfully we make use of our middle years and beyond.

At 40-plus, we have choices: we can go into mourning for our lost youth and opportunities, or we can see it as second-chance time.

It is not too late to increase our fitness and improve the healthiness of our diet, and to take in general a more proactive, self-help approach to maximising our health. For example, we can still benefit enormously from giving up smoking if we haven't yet done so, or from becoming more resolute in avoiding passive smoking if we have. We can still periodically take out our attitudes and beliefs and dust them down. Can the evidence at hand and our experience still support them? Or are we operating on an anachronistic set of prejudices without even realising how they are limiting our choices in life?

We can reassess our ways of recognising and dealing with sources of stress in our lives and, when they are no longer serving us well, change them. And far from being trapped in an immutable psychological straightjacket, we can certainly still discover new and more positive ways to react to change and challenge. We can learn to let go; to refuse to allow the present and the future to be chained to the past.

The years after 40 can be a time when new opportunities

present themselves to us. All we need is to be open enough to recognise and brave enough to grab them. Many of us find ourselves at 40 and beyond with more time and money, post young child-rearing, to pay a little more attention to ourselves; to put more energy and effort into our careers; to discover and meet our own needs. And many seem to be appreciating it.

A survey published by the marketing organisation Mintel in November 1993 found that people aged between 50 and 64 spend more money each week than any other age group (£124 a head), with 30-to-49-year-olds runners up (£112) and under-30s bringing up the rear (£107). In addition, it found today's 50-somethings 'the happiest and healthiest' as well as 'the wealthiest' that this age group has ever been in this century. Angela Hughes, Mintel's consumer research manager, said when the report was published, 'Whatever might be said about youth or your schooldays being the best time of your life, those who have lived a bit longer clearly think otherwise.'

There may be some physical prizes we are unlikely to win post-40, but even in areas where youth once reigned supreme the middle-aged are beginning to make a challenge. Take the case of Lauren Hutton, the model who at age 51 is beating the pants off most younger rivals. In 1993, 20 years after signing a £200,000-a-year-contract to promote a cosmetics range – a deal that made her the first of the 'super-models' – she signed a considerably greater 'mega-contract' with the same company. It turned on its head the tradition of using girls too young to need them to sell expensive cosmetics to women motivated enough by encroaching wrinkles to buy them. And it worked. Women past 40 were so inspired by pictures of someone their own age in the advertisements to buy the products that they bought and bought – and the company has now branched out into a whole new skin-care range specifically for those beyond the first flush.

Even more encouragingly, Hutton, who has refused the aid of plastic surgery to protect her valuable financial assets, negotiated her own deal and included in it a clause that her photographs would not be retouched. 'I don't want to look like an egg,' she said. 'My face used to be airbrushed to death. I don't want it to be any more.'

Conspicuous late developers – such as best-selling author Mary

Wesley, who was 70 when she published the first of her nine novels, and Winston Churchill, who was a mere 65 when he took the helm as wartime leader in 1940 – may be more exception than rule. But the shrinking jobs market and the accelerating rate of technological change are forcing more and more of us into a mid-life change of direction whether we like it or not. For many, that will mean second careers, some with notable success in them. Others may find, second time round, the satisfaction of getting to do something they really enjoy, either in the job market or out of it – possibly something we would never have considered trying when we were younger.

One way to maximise our chances of enjoying the 40-plus years is to have a positive attitude towards the possibilities in them – and in ourselves. We may even feel like thumbing our noses at the reverence for youth and the supremacy of the youth culture that so dominated recent decades. At 40 onwards, we may have a few more bulges and lines than we want, but we also have the invaluable assets of maturity and the experience we have gained of life. Once we learn to understand and value those, others will begin to respond to those resources, and to us, in the same way.

Such an attitude towards age has been promoted quite assertively on the other side of the Atlantic, where the Grey Panther movement became an important political lobby by constantly reminding politicians how great a proportion of the population is now past the first flush – but still alive and voting.

Where Grey Panther led, Grey Pride followed. The American women who hang from their office walls the defiant signal, 'I don't have hot flashes, I have power surges,' are also contributing to a growing confidence that 40-plus is not synonymous with 'somewhat past it'.

Opportunities

No previous generation post-40 has had the opportunities open to us for new and varied leisure activities, to do voluntary work, and for continuing to learn and to train.

Later learning
The older we are, the less likely we are to have had the educational

opportunities, first time round, we could expect if we were young today. 'The great majority of older people had little initial schooling,' say Tom Schuller and Anne Marie Bostyn in *Learning: Education, Training and Information in The Third Age***, one of the research papers published by the Carnegie Inquiry into The Third Age. (The inquiry defined the third age as 50 to 74.)

They continue: 'Roughly two in three people over 50 and under the state pension age (60/65) left school at 15 or earlier, compared with one in four of those under 50. This initial disadvantage has not been corrected by subsequent education.'

The inquiry found that the distribution of educational opportunity was both gender- and class-related. Although women's initial schooling was only slightly shorter, their level of qualification remains significantly lower. And nearly nine out of ten unskilled or semi-skilled workers have no qualifications at all. 'Each succeeding generation,' the authors found, 'is better educated than its predecessor, as measured by length of initial schooling and possession of formal qualifications.'

If we over-40s have tended to be relative education have-nots first time round, we now have a wide range of opportunities to go back to learning with whatever level of commitment suits us. Whether you are looking for an evening class in vegetarian cookery or a higher degree in an abstruse area of quantum physics, chances are you will find it if you shop around.

Adult education institutes and further education colleges offer a wide range of day and evening classes all over the country. Your local library should have details of those close to you. Options include access courses to enable people to gain qualifications for college entry. If cost is a concern, they usually offer reduced rates for the unwaged.

Some universities and colleges run courses for members of the public in the evenings or during holidays. Some also offer diploma or degree courses part-time, which enable you to study for a qualification over a number of years.

One of the great success stories of adult education has been the Open University*, which opened its doors to its first 24,000 students in 1971. Since then, 122,500 people have graduated and the O.U. now has more students than any other British university. In 1993, it had more than 220,000 students on its books, 4000 of whom were resident outside the UK. Nearly 130,000 were studying for a first or higher degree, or studying a single subject from a degree programme, or were on a short course. And more than 82,000 more had bought self-contained study packs to work through on their own or in groups.

The majority of O.U. students are in their 20s, 30s or 40s. The youngest are in their late teens and the oldest graduates to date have been in their 90s. Almost half are women – a higher proportion than at any other UK university. The O.U. has undergraduate and higher degree programmes as well as courses in manufacturing and computing, professional development in education, health and social welfare, community education and leisure studies. The next major academic development is to be modern languages, not for beginners but for people who want to take school-level language skills to a more advanced stage.

The O.U. academic year runs from February to October for those in degree programmes, and there are no educational prerequisites for entry. People usually spread getting a degree over four to eight years.

Students study mostly at home and in their own time. Written course work is backed up by tutor feedback and a system of local tutorials through a network of 250 study centres (availability depends on course popularity and population-centre size). There are also television and radio broadcasts and audio and video cassettes. Some courses also involve home experiment kits, home computing and short residential summer schools, held on university campuses during their summer vacations.

Fees are around £270 a course for undergraduates and another £180 if there is a summer school. At 1993 prices, the O.U. reckons you can expect to pay about £2,500 to obtain a degree. There is a student hardship fund for people who have difficulty meeting the cost, and payment can be by instalment.

Following the success of the Open University came the Open College of the Arts★, which is now affiliated with the O.U. The full implications of the new relationship for academic recognition of Open College courses had, at early 1994, yet to be worked out. Students who complete a course with the Open College get a Record of Satisfactory Completion and can ask for a graded award if they want written evidence of their level of achievement.

Courses, which consist of practical work, tutor feedback, and further tutorial support through around 100 local tutorial centres, can include subjects such as creative writing, art appreciation, sculpture, music, art and design, painting, garden design, video and textiles.

Prices range from £155 for a course on drawing that would take about five months working three or four hours a week on it, to £315 for a first-level course in garden design which assumes no previous knowledge and after which a student can follow up with a second-level course. Some subjects, such as painting, can be studied at a third level, too.

There are also numerous colleges offering correspondence courses on almost any subject you can think of – and a few that may never have occurred to you. One of the best-known is the National Extension College*, a non-profit-making organisation which offers GCSEs and A levels, and courses leading to City and Guilds Certificates and National Vocational Qualifications.

It has study-skill courses and courses to prepare you for under-graduate study; many people use the NEC as a route into the Open University. The NEC also offers tuition towards a degree with London University, towards certificates and diplomas with the Institute of Linguists, and for Engineering Council examinations. There are nearly 100 topics on offer, ranging from accounting to zoo-animal management, as well as counselling, editing, Gaelic, numeracy skills, self-employment, Welsh and voluntary work.

The NEC teaches by a mixture of written and taped material, and you have a personal tutor. Fees per subject start at £60 and go up to £365. GCSEs and A levels come cheaper if you buy in bulk. One A level is £235, for example, but you can do three for £625. There are discounts for low-earners and an instalment plan for spreading payment.

You can get tax relief on some vocational courses, and your local Training Enterprise Council* may be able to pay part of the fee for a vocational course. Or you may be eligible for a Career Development Loan (CDL) of between £200 and £5000 for up to 80 per cent of fees; you would not have to repay the loan until three months after the end of your course. To find out if you are eligible for a CDL, contact the Employment Department, Career Development Loans Unit*.

For a list of other accredited colleges offering correspondence courses, or to check out the validity of the qualification you will get at the end of any correspondence course of study you are considering doing, contact the Council for the Accreditation of Correspondence Colleges*.

New activities

If you want to find the nearest group of people who share an interest or undertake an activity in which you are interested, look for information in your local newspaper or library. There is also an excellent book published by the National Council of Voluntary Organisations called *The Voluntary Agencies Directory*★★, which is regularly revised and provides details of headquarters and local branches of all sorts of groups, from those offering help and support to people with a particular problem, to groups who come together to share the same hobby or pleasure.

If you cannot find the right group for you, consider starting one. You might find some helpful ideas on getting it off the ground in the book *How to Raise Funds and Sponsorship: A Complete Step-by-step Guide to Success*★★ by Chriss McCallum. Another useful publication is *Self-help Groups: Getting Started; Keeping Going*★★ by Judy Wilson. It has a bias towards setting up self-help groups for people who share serious personal problems. But some of its sensible suggestions would be equally relevant to setting up any interest group.

Volunteering

People who do voluntary work find it can provide them with a range of satisfactions, including widening their social networks and interests, substituting for paid work during unemployment or post-retirement, and providing a sense of self-worth and of being of value in their communities.

Some voluntary work also provides free training. For example, the Samaritans*, the marriage guidance organisation Relate* and the bereavement charity Cruse* all give training in counselling to those who get through their tough selection procedures.

Many charities now accept that volunteers should be repaid out-of-pocket expenses. If money is tight, don't be deterred by fears that giving your time could also cost you money.

REASONS FOR VOLUNTEERING

According to the 1991 National Survey of Voluntary Activity in the UK (see Recommended Reading on p. 220), the reason people give for volunteering change slightly at different ages.

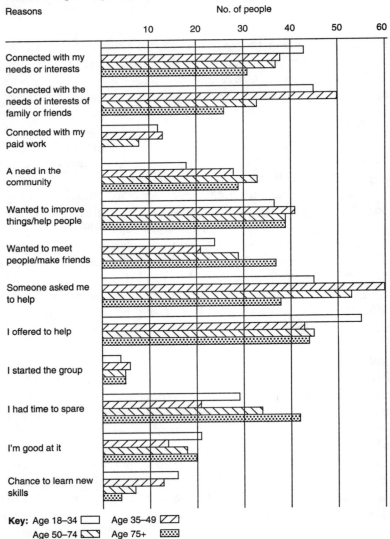

Reasons   No. of people

Key: Age 18–34   Age 35–49
        Age 50–74   Age 75+

How people found the voluntary organisation to which they give time was also been studied by a MORI** survey in 1990. Table 1 sums up what it found, and may give you some ideas if you are looking for an organisation or group to whom you can volunteer your time. Talking to relatives and friends and reading the local paper may point you in the right direction. Churches, schools, charity shops and hospitals also often need helpers.

The *Voluntary Agencies Directory* mentioned in the previous section is also a useful source of information. Entries for every one of the organisations listed say whether they want volunteers, as well as giving a headquarters address. Or, if you look in your local phone book under 'volunteer', you should find any volunteer bureaux or volunteer co-ordinating centres operating in your area. Your council and library should know about them, too.

Volunteering can, of course, mean anything from putting in a few hours a month with a local group to putting your normal life on hold and doing a two-year stint abroad with someone like Voluntary Service Overseas*. (But don't expect to come home and pick up where you left off. You are unlikely to remain unchanged by the experience.)

VSO accepts volunteers aged from 20 to 70 without dependent children who can back up their practical expertise with some

Table 1: HOW I FIRST BECAME INVOLVED IN VOLUNTEERING

Route	Overall	35-54	55 +
Through friend	34	31	36
Through relative	32	38	25
By first being a member	24	29	30
Through work	22	25	15
Following a leaflet drop	4	3	3
Volunteer bureau	3	3	5
Advert in local press	3	3	2
Advert in national press	2	2	1
Newsletter	2	1	1
Local library	1	1	1
National radio	3	1	–
Base	598	207	195

Figures are percentages of volunteers who got involved through the particular route.
Source: MORI survvey 1990.

paper qualifications, who want to work in the Third World and who are willing to do so for a local salary. The organisation attempts to meet requests from developing countries for people who can offer training in a range of subjects from agriculture – through business, education, health care, journalism, social work, teaching and so on – to zoological research. People with experience in teaching sport, as librarians, or of secretarial work (even if they have only basic training in shorthand and typing) are particularly in demand at present.

Dozens of other organisations do voluntary work abroad. Most of them positively encourage the over-40s, for the life experience they bring with them. There are several books which might help you to find the right one for you. Try *International Directory of Voluntary Work*★★ by David Woodworth, *Directory of Work and Study in Developing Countries*★★, or *Volunteer Work*★★ by Hilary Sewell. Or contact the Central Bureau for Educational Visits and Exchanges★ for information and details of other publications.

If you feel you have skills to impart but want to do it closer to home, you might find your input would be appreciated by a local jobs club (find one via your local authority or library) or youth club. Or you could start a learning group of your own. (See section on New activities, above, for hints on how to go about it.)

Another outlet for your knowledge and ability if you want to volunteer them might be the University of the Third Age★, or U3A, an umbrella organisation which co-ordinates the activities of more than 100 local groups around the country. These local groups offer talks, study groups, travel opportunities etc. mainly for the retired but also for the unemployed. Members decide their own programmes and set their own fees. There is a help pack called U3A DIY available for people who want to set up a local U3A, and a magazine, *The Third Age*, gives details of conferences and events.

Goal planning

One way to increase our chances of achieving greater satisfaction – whatever that may mean to us – for ourselves in the second half of our lives is to invest time in planning our goals. We are far more likely to get the things we most want out of life if we take the time and trouble to discover what they are.

One way to become clearer about them is to work at deciding our goals, and then at revising them from time to time. To do it, we need to make a list of the things we would like to have achieved in three months, in six months, in a year, in two years, in five years and ten years from now. We need to make sure that we cover all the areas of our lives that are important to us. These may include career, leisure, health and fitness, personal relationships, personal growth, spiritual growth, financial security or advancement.

To increase our chances for success, here are some rules to follow:

- **Each goal should be specific.** For example, it is too vague to say you want to be at the top of your career in 10 years' time. A specific goal might be that you want to be managing director of a firm of which you are the owner in 10 years' time.
- **Work out some intermediate steps** once you have established specific long-term goals.
- **Make your goals measurable.** 'Being rich' in five years' time is not measurable. Earning £X a year, or the then equivalent of £X now, is.
- **Ensure that your goals are achievable.** Owning a four-bedroomed home in five years' time may be. Owning a home on the moon is not. Setting impossible goals can be a way people set themselves up to fail.
- **Be sure that your goals are compatible with your personal sense of responsibility.** If we set goals that are not compatible with our personal 'ecology' or would be damaging to our relationships or to those around us, we would be ambivalent about achieving them and unlikely to allow ourselves to do so.

Once you have worked out your goals, record them in a notebook or diary and take them out again once every few months to review your progress. Revise them if need be.

Having and keeping in touch with written goals clarifies our thinking, helps us identify our priorities, makes us more likely to spot opportunities when they come our way. Goal-planning, in short, increases the chances that we will achieve what we want out of life — at 40 and beyond.

ANSWERS TO QUIZ

1. a through h. Diet is related to all of them.

2. b. The average aerobic capacity of the fittest 10 per cent of men aged 65 to 74 is higher, according to research, than that of the least-fit 10 per cent of men aged 25 to 34. Thus a fit man of 74 may well have more 'puff' than an unfit 25-year-old. The pattern for women is much the same.

3. b. Best-selling author Mary Wesley was 70 when she published the first of her nine novels. Churchill was a mere 65 when he took the helm as wartime leader in 1940.

4. a. Research now suggests it is not just a matter of how much excess weight we have, but also where we wear it – whether we are pear-shaped or apple-shaped. Being overweight poses a bigger health threat if we are the apple shape that many chubby men have (and which often indicates a high level of cholesterol in the blood) than if the excess comes to roost more on the hips, in the pear shape more usual for over-weight women.

5. e. A study by Richard Peto, reported in *The Lancet* in 1992, reckoned that one smoker in three dies of smoking-related diseases. And this was just one of a number of recent studies to have arrived at similar figures.

6. b. When *Which?* magazine investigated slimming products, it found that the 13 meal replacements assessed were often high in fat, sugar and calories and only one plan could show the researchers proof of long-term success. So the answer is – £££s.

7. b. Long-term passive smoking increases the risk for non-smokers of lung cancer from 10 per cent to 30 per cent – or by a factor of two – according to recent research.

8. a. Studies show that one woman in ten after the age of 70 will in a five-year period suffer a hip fracture due, at least in part, to osteoporosis, or the weakening of the bone because of calcium loss. And many women with osteoporosis have several fractures.

9. b. It is estimated that 75 per cent of illnesses reported to GPs are stress–related.

Useful addresses

Here are the details of organisations that have been marked with an asterisk in the text. Most expect or appreciate a large stamped and self-addressed envelope in which to reply to enquiries. It also helps if you include your telephone number, so they can contact you if they are unclear about how best they can help you. Some organisations make a charge for a copy of their directory of members.

CHAPTER 2

Health Education Authority, HEA Business Unit, Christchurch College, North Holmes Road, Canterbury, Kent CT1 IQU; telephone (0227) 455564.

Ramblers' Association, 1-5 Wandsworth Road, London SW8 2XX; telephone 071-582 6878.

Regional offices of the **Sports Council**:
East Midlands, covers Derbyshire, Nottinghamshire, Lincolnshire, Leicestershire and Northamptonshire; telephone (0602) 821887.
Eastern Region, covers Bedfordshire, Hertfordshire, Cambridgeshire, Suffolk, Norfolk and Essex; telephone (0234) 345222.
Greater London and South-east, covers greater London, Surrey, Kent and East and West Sussex; telephone 081-778 8600.
North-west, covers Lancashire, Cheshire, greater Manchester and Merseyside; telephone 061-834 0338.
Northern, covers Northumberland, Cumbria, Durham, Cleveland, Tyne and Wear; telephone 091-384 9595.
South-west, covers Avon, Cornwall, Devon, Dorset, Somerset, Wiltshire and Gloucestershire; telephone (0460) 73491.

Southern, covers Hampshire, Isle of Wight, Berkshire, Buckinghamshire and Oxfordshire; telephone (0734) 483311.
West Midlands, covers the West Midlands, Hereford and Worcester, Shropshire, Staffordshire and Warwickshire; telephone 021-456 3444.
Yorkshire and Humberside, covers West, South and North Yorkshire and Humberside; telephone (0532) 436443.
Sports Council for Wales; telephone (0222) 397571.
Sports Council for Northern Ireland; telephone (0232) 381222.
Scottish Sports Council; telephone 031-317 7200.

CHAPTER 4

Council for Acupuncture, 179 Gloucester Place, London NW1 6BX; telephone 071-724 5756.

British Acupuncture Association, 34 Alderney Street, London SW1V 4EU; telephone 071-834 1012.

Traditional Acupuncture Society, 1 The Ridgeway, Stratford upon Avon, Warwickshire CV37 9JL; telephone (0789) 298789.

Quit, 102 Gloucester Place, London W1H 3DA; **Quitline** telephone helpline open Monday to Friday 9.30am to 5.30pm on 071-487 3000.

National Council of Psychotherapists and Hypnotherapy Register, 24 Rickmansworth Road, Watford, Hertfordshire WD1 7HT; telephone (0923) 227772.

Institute for Complementary Medicine, PO Box 194, London SE16 1QZ.

Alcohol Concern, 275 Gray's Inn Road, London WC1X 8QF; telephone 071-833 3471.

Alcoholics Anonymous, General Service Office, PO Box 1, Stonebow House, Stonebow, York YO1 2NJ; telephone (0904) 644026. Or look under Alcohol in your local telephone directory.

Al-Anon, 61 Great Dover Street, London SE1 4YF; telephone 071-403 0888 – 24-hour confidential help line.

Alateen, as Al-Anon above.

CHAPTER 5

Relate, Herbert Gray College, Little Church Street, Rugby, Warwickwickshire CV21 3AP; telephone (0788) 573241. Or look in your local telephone directory.

National Childbirth Trust, Alexandra House, Oldham Terrace, Acton, London W3 6NH; telephone 081-992 8637.

CHAPTER 6

Arthritis and Rheumatism Council, Copeman House, St Mary's Court, St Mary's Gate, Chesterfield, Derbyshire S41 7TD; telephone (0246) 558033.

British Chiropractic Association, 29 Whitley Street, Reading, Berkshire RG2 0EG.

British Homoeopathic Association, 27a Devonshire Street, London WIN 1RJ; telephone 071-935 2163.

Society of Homoeopaths, 2 Artizan Road, Northampton NN1 4HU; telephone (0604) 21400.

General Council and Register of Osteopaths, 56 London Road, Reading, Berkshire RG1 4SQ; telephone (0734) 576585.

Chartered Society of Physiotherapy, 14 Bedford Row, London WC1R 4ED; telephone 071-242 1941.

Organisation of Chartered Physiotherapists in Private Practice, Suite 8, Weston Chambers, Weston Road, Southend-on-Sea, Essex SS1 1AT; telephone (0702) 392124.

CHAPTER 7

MIND, Granta House, 15-19 Broadway, Stratford, London E15 4BQ; telephone 081-519 2122.

Citizens Advice Bureaux, National Association of Citizens Advice Bureaux Central Office, Myddelton House, 115-123 Pentonville Road, London N1 9LZ; telephone 071-833 2181. Or look in your local telephone directory for your local office.

Victim Support, Cranmer House, 39 Brixton Road, London SW9 6DD; telephone 071-735 9166. Or look in your local telephone directory.

Council for Acupuncture, see under Chapter 4.

British Acupuncture Association, see under Chapter 4.

Traditional Acupuncture Society, see under Chapter 4.

Society of Teachers of the Alexander Technique, 20 London House, 266 Fulham Road, London SW10 9EL; telephone 071-351 0828.

International Federation of Aromatherapists, Department of Continuing Education, Royal Masonic Hospital, Ravenscourt Park, London W6 OTN. (The directory of qualified aromatherapists costs £2 – s.a.e. required.)

British Association for Autogenic Training and Therapy, 86 Harley Street, London W1N 1AE.

British Holistic Medical Association, 179 Gloucester Place, London NW1 6DX; telephone 071-262 5299.

British Complementary Medicine Association, St Charles Hospital, Exmoor Street, London W10 6DZ; telephone 081-964 1205.

Stresswise, PO Box 5, Congleton, Cheshire CW12 1XE.

Institute for Complementary Medicine, see under Chapter 4.

National Council of Psychotherapists and Hypnotherapy Register, see under Chapter 4.

British Association for Counselling, 1 Regent Place, Rugby, Warwickshire CV21 2PJ; telephone (0788) 578328.

Relate, see under Chapter 5.

Cruse Bereavement Care, Cruse House, 126 Sheen Road, Richmond, Surrey TW9 1UR; telephone 081-940 4818.

British Massage Therapy Council, 3 Woodhouse Cliff, Headingley, Leeds, West Yorkshire LS6 2HF; telephone (0532) 785601.

Transcendental Meditation, Freepost, London SW1P 4YY; telephone Freephone (0800) 269303.

Chartered Society of Physiotherapy, see under Chapter 6.

Organisation of Chartered Physiotherapists in Private Practice, see under Chapter 6.

United Kingdom Council of Psychotherapists, Regent's College, Inner Circle, Regent's Park, London NW1 4NS; telephone 071-487 7554.

British Association for Counselling, see above.

Institute for Complementary Medicine, see under Chapter 4.

British School of Reflexology, 92 Sheering Road, Old Harlow, Essex CM17 0JW; telephone (0279) 429060.

The Shiatsu Society, 5 Foxcote, Wokingham, Berkshire RG11 3PG; telephone (0734) 730836.

British T'ai Chi Chuan Centre, Unit C, Maybanks House, Maybanks Road, South Woodford, London E18; telephone 081-502 9307.

Wheel of Yoga, 1 Hamilton Place, Boston Road, Sleaford, Lincolnshire NG34 7ES; telephone (0529) 306851.

CHAPTER 8

Open University, PO Box 200, Walton Hall, Milton Keynes, MK7 6YZ; telephone (0908) 653231.

Open College of the Arts, Houndhill, Worsbrough, Barnsley, South Yorkshire S70 6TU; telephone (0226) 730495.

National Extension College, 18 Brooklands Avenue, Cambridge CB2 2HN; telephone (0223) 316644.

Training Enterprise Councils are run by the Department of Employment. Find your nearest via your local Jobcentre.

Employment Department, Career Development Loans Unit, Room 359, Caxton House, Tothill Street, London SW1H 9NF; telephone (0800) 585 505.

Council for the Accreditation of Correspondence Colleges, 27 Marylebone Road, London NW1 5JS; telephone 071-935 5391.

National Council of Voluntary Organisations, Regents Wharf, 8 All Saints Street, London N1 9RL; telephone 071-713 6161.

The Samaritans, 10 The Grove, Slough, Berkshire SL1 1QP; telephone (0753) 532713. Or look in your local telephone directory.

Relate, see under Chapter 5.

Cruse, see under Chapter 7.

Voluntary Service Overseas, 317 Putney Bridge Road, London SW15 2PN; telephone 071-780 2266.

Central Bureau for Educational Visits and Exchanges, Seymour Mews House, Seymour Mews, London W1H 9PE; telephone 071-486 5101.

University of the Third Age, U3A National Office, 1 Stockwell Green, London SW9 9JS; telephone 071-737 2541.

Recommended reading

Further details of books that have been recommended and marked in the text with a double asterisk are given below.

CHAPTER 1

Understanding Back Trouble, a Which? Consumer Guide published by Consumers' Association and Hodder & Stoughton.

CHAPTER 2

Soft Exercise: Complete Book of Stretching by Arthur Balaskas and John Stirk, published by Unwin Paperbacks.

CHAPTER 3

Which? Way to a Healthier Diet by Judy Byrne, a Which? Consumer Guide published by Consumers' Association and Hodder and Stoughton.

CHAPTER 5

The Which? Guide to Men's Health by Dr Steve Carroll, a Which? Consumer Guide published by Consumers' Association.
The National Childbirth Trust Book of Pregnancy, Birth and Parenthood edited by Glynnis Tucker, published by Oxford Paperbacks.
Better Late than Never: Becoming an Older Mother by Maggie Jones, to be published by Optima in January 1995.
Understanding HRT and the Menopause by Dr Robert C.D. Wilson, a Which? Consumer Guide published by Consumers' Association and Hodder and Stoughton.
Menopause without Medicine by Linda Ojeda, published by Thorsons.

CHAPTER 6

Understanding Back Trouble, a Which? Consumer Guide published by Consumers' Association and Hodder & Stoughton.
Preventing Heart Disease by the Coronary Prevention Group, a Which? Consumer Guide published by Consumers' Association and Hodder &

Stoughton. (There is also a video, 'You can prevent heart disease', produced by Consumers' Association in conjunction with the British Heart Foundation.)

CHAPTER 7

Feeling Good – The New Mood Therapy by David D. Burns, published by Signet.

The Feeling Good Handbook by David D. Burns, published by Plume.

A Woman in Your Own Right – Assertiveness and You by Anne Dickson, published by Quartet.

Self-hypnosis: The Complete Manual for Health and Self-change by Brian M. Alman and Peter T. Lambrou, published by Souvenir Press.

Understanding Stress, a Which? Consumer Guide published by Consumers' Association and Hodder & Stoughton.

CHAPTER 8

Learning: Education, Training and Information in The Third Age by Tom Schuller and Anne Marie Bostyn. This is Research Paper No. 3 of the Carnegie Inquiry into The Third Age and is published by the Carnegie United Kingdom Trust.

The Voluntary Agencies Directory 93/94, published by NCVO Publications.

How to Raise Funds and Sponsorship: A Complete Step-by-step Guide to Success by Chriss McCallum, published by How To Books, Plymouth.

Self-help Groups: Getting Started; Keeping Going by Judy Wilson is a Longman Self-help guide.

The 1991 National Survey of Voluntary Activity in the UK, Voluntary Action Research Second Series, Paper No. 1 by P. Lynn and J. Davis Smith, Volunteer Centre UK, Berkhamsted.

Voluntary Activity: A Survey of Public Attitudes, MORI, the Volunteer Centre, UK.

International Directory of Voluntary Work by David Woodworth, published by Vacation-Work, Oxford.

Directory of Work and Study in Developing Countries, published by Vacation-Work, Oxford.

Volunteer Work Abroad by Hilary Sewell, from the Central Bureau for Educational Visits and Exchanges.

Other publications you might find helpful include:

Fifty Plus Lifeguide by Dr Miriam Stoppard, published by Dorling Kindersley.

Health Wise, An Intelligent Guide for the Over Sixties by James Le Fanu, published by Papermac.

INDEX

acupuncture 102–3, 190–1
addictions 190
adrenaline 168
aerobics 41–2, 54–5, 61
ageing process 7, 11, 176–7
alcohol
    hangovers 106
    health risks 105–6
    heart disease and 104–5
    moderate drinking 104, 105,
        106–7
    recommended upper limits 107–8
    reducing consumption 107
    self-help groups 108
Alexander Technique 191
amniocentesis 117–18
anaemia 79
angina 23, 62, 148
ankylosing spondylitis 137
antioxidants 73–4
anxiety 190, 192, 196
aqua-aerobics 41–2
aromatherapy 191–2
arthritis 20, 56, 153–4, 155–6, 194
    see also osteo; rheumatoid
aspirin 149–50, 158
assertiveness training 183–4
asthma 56, 94, 95, 190, 191, 194
atherosclerosis 85, 148
autogenic training 192

back problems 27, 46–7, 56, 137–9,
        160, 194, 196
badminton 42, 60
biofeedback 192–3
bladder problems 122, 130
body
    bones 19
    cartilage 20
    heart 21–3
    joints 19
    knees 20
    ligaments 19
    lungs 23–4
    muscles 20–21
    skeleton 19–20
    spine 137–8
    tendons 19
body mass index (BMI) 88
bone mass loss 14, 80, 125, 154–5
    see also osteoporosis
bowel problems 66, 70
bowls 42
breast cancer 14, 129, 141, 142–3
breasts
    changes in 125
    self-examination 144–5
breathing techniques 23, 187–8
breathlessness 18
brittle bones see osteoporosis
bronchitis 56, 94, 190

caffeine consumption 108–11
calcium 77, 79–81
calorie consumption 11
cancer
    age and associated risk of 140
    detection 142–6
    diet and 66, 73, 74, 140
    fitness and 14
    preventive measures 140–2
    smoking and 94, 96, 98, 141
    see also types of
cartilage 20
cell renewal 7
cervical smear tests 142
cervix, cancer of the 140
chiropractic 159–60
cholesterol
    caffeine intake and 109–10
    and heart disease 84–5, 86, 109–10
    reducing blood levels 14, 70, 87

sources 84, 85
tests 86–7
circuit training 42–3
clinical hypnosis 193
co-ordination 14
coffee and tea drinking 91, 108–11
cognitive therapy 182, 196
constipation 70, 107, 194
counselling 193
cramp 194
crime, fear of 182–3
cross–training 16, 61
cycling 39, 43–5

dancing 45
dental disease 66, 69
depression 88, 190, 196
diabetes 14, 66, 130
diet 62, 65–6, 81, 89, 130–1, 140
diverticular disease 70
dowager's hump 155
Down's syndrome 117–18
educational opportunities
    Career Development Loan (CDL)
        206
    correspondence courses 206–7
    National Extension College 206
    Open College of the Arts 205–6
    Open University 204–5
    University of the Third Age 210
elderly people
    caring for 175
    vitamin deficiencies 75
emphysema 24, 94
endometriosis 129, 130, 141
exercise
    anti-exercise lobby 13
    benefits 8, 14, 16, 158
    breathing patterns 23
    checking with your doctor 37, 38
    clothing 27
    dehydration 24
    during the menopause 131–2
    injuries 19, 26–7
    local authority sports facilities 38
    moderate/vigorous 19
    protection against illness 13–14,
        16–17, 62–3
    pulse rate and 21, 24–6
    regular commitment 17, 62

sports shoes 54, 59–62
exercise bikes 44–5
exercise classes 46, 61
exercise programmes
    activity ratings 40
    before you start 26–8
    choosing the best activity 37
    cross–training 16, 61
    exercising safely 38–9
    Kegel exercises 115, 122, 124
    stretching exercises 28–35
    videos 57–8
    warming up and cooling down 27
    see also types of activity

fats
    essential fatty acids 72
    monounsaturates 70, 71
    polyunsaturates 70, 71
    recommended limits 67–8
    saturated fats 68, 70, 71, 82, 86
female menopause
    benefits of exercise 131–2
    bone mass loss 125
    cardiovascular changes 125–6
    dietary advice 130–1
    duration 118
    life style 132
    menstrual cycle and 119–21
    minimising the effects of 130–2
    peri-menopause 121
    psychological impact 113, 126
    sexual difficulties 115
    smoking and 94
    symptoms 122, 124–6
        see also hormone replacement
        therapy (HRT); osteoporosis
fibre 67, 69–70
fibrositis 20
fitness
    aerobic fitness 15, 16
    age and activity targets 18, 19
    age and fitness levels 11–12
    components of 15–16, 39
    facts 14
    fitness test 24–5
    good health and 12
    and mortality rates 17
    national survey 12–13, 18–19
    personal perceptions of 12–13

stamina 15
strength 15–16
suppleness 15, 28
see also exercise; exercise
    programmes
fractures 190
further education *see* educational
    opportunities

gall bladder disease 130
gallstones 14, 66
gangrene 94
goal planning 210–11
golf 46–7, 199
gout 14
grandparenting 175–6

headaches 190, 191, 192, 194, 196
health clubs and gyms 39, 48–9
health problems
    alternative medicine 159–63
    role of exercise 158
    specific disorders 137–58
healthy eating
    carbohydrates 66–7, 69
    changing your diet 65–6
    cholesterol 84–7
    and disease prevention 66, 74, 140
    during the menopause 130–1
    fat 67–8, 70–2, 82
    fibre 67, 69–70
    food preparation 82–3
    fruit and vegetables 66, 74
    guidelines 66–8, 81–3
    menu planning 83–4
    minerals and trace elements 75–81
    oils 70, 71, 72, 82
    protein 68, 72
    salt 68, 72–3, 78, 81
    shopping for food 81–2
    sugar 69, 81
    vitamins and vitamin supplements
        73–5
    wholemeal foods 67
    see also weight control
heart disease
    alcohol consumption and 104–5
        angina 23, 62, 148
    benefits of exercise 13–14, 17, 23,
        62

cholesterol and 84–5, 86, 109–10
diet and 66, 73, 74
heart attacks 14, 17, 23, 93, 148–
    9, 177–8, 192
heart–valve disease 149
main types of 147–9
personality types and 177–8
reducing risk of 149–50
smoking and 92–3, 95, 98
women and 125–6, 146–7
heart rate 21, 23, 26, 27
hiatus hernia 14, 190
high blood pressure *see* hypertension
hiking 49–50
hip replacements 153–4
home fitness equipment 44–5, 50–1
homoeopathy 160–1
hormone replacement therapy
    (HRT)
    background 127
    benefits 128–9
    cancer and 129, 141
    drawbacks 129, 130
    protection against bone loss 80,
        81, 125, 129, 155
    protection against heart disease
        150
    smokers and 130
    techniques 127–8
hot flushes 124, 131, 132
hypertension 14, 27, 66, 110, 150–2,
    158
hyperventilation 187
hypnosis 103–4, 193, 197
hypnotherapy 193

impotence 114–15
incontinence 122
indigestion 190
insomnia 131, 152–3, 188, 192, 194,
    196
intestinal problems 66, 70
iron 77, 79
irritable bowel syndrome 70

jogging 47–8, 60
joint pains 37, 55–6
joint replacement surgery 153–4,
    156

keep-fit classes 51, 61
kidney disease 110, 137, 151
knee injuries 20

leukaemia 94
life style, stress and 174–5, 181
lipoproteins 71, 85, 86
liver disease 130
looking forward
  educational opportunities 203–7
  goal planning 210–11
  late developers 202–3
  new activities 207
    opportunities and challenges
    201–3.
  voluntary work 207–10
lumbago 20
lung cancer 92, 94, 95, 98

magnesium 78
male menopause
  coping with 134–5
  sexual difficulties 115, 133–4
  symptoms 133
  testosterone therapy treatment
    114, 133
malignant melanoma 141
mammograms 142–3
massage 193–4
meditation 170, 194–5
men
  impotence 114–15
  male menopause 115, 132–5
  osteoporosis 80
menopause see female menopause;
    male menopause
mental health 8
  see also stress
metabolism 24
migraine 190, 192, 196
minerals and trace elements
  calcium 77, 79–81
  functions and sources 76–7
  iron 77, 79
  magnesium 78
  selenium 78
  zinc 77, 79
muscle relaxation 194–5
muscles
  exercise and 20–1

muscle strength 15–16, 20, 21
  types of 20

nausea 110
neuralgia 190, 191
nicotine 95–6, 98
night sweats 124, 132

obesity 14, 66, 87–8, 97, 190
oestrogen 80, 120–2, 124–5, 129,
    141
  see also hormone replacement
    therapy (HRT)
orienteering 51–2
osteoarthritis 14, 59, 153–4, 190,
    191
osteopathy 159, 161–2
osteoporosis
  benefits of exercise 14, 56
  changes in bone mass 80, 125,
    154–5
  diet and 66, 79–81
  smoking and 94
ovarian cancer 129

pain, stress and 171–2
palpitations 110, 124, 131
panic attacks 110
peptic ulcers 94
personal safety 183
personal trainers 52
physiotherapy 162–3, 195
polluted air 43–4
posture 15, 16
power walking 52–3
pre-menstrual syndrome 110
pregnancy
  after 40 116–18
  smoking during 95
protein 68, 72
psychotherapy 195–6
pulse rate 21, 24–6

quiz: fit and healthy at 40+ 10

reflexology 196
rehearsal techniques 196–7
reproductive system 122
respiration 23–4
retirement 176, 181

rheumatoid arthritis 155–6, 190
rowing machines 51
running 53–4

sciatica 20
selenium 78, 140
self-defence 183
self-hypnosis 197
sexual problems
    declining sex drive 133–4
    impotence 114–15
    menopausal 115, 133
    seeking help 116
    stress–related 116, 134, 165
sexual relations 113–14
shiatsu 197
sight, loss of 151
single people 176
skin cancer 141–2
skin and hair changes 124
skipping ropes 51
sleep problems 131, 152–3, 188–9,
    192, 194, 196
slimming diets 89
smoking
    and cancer 94, 96, 98, 141
    children of smokers 95
    cigarette smoke 95–6
    and coronary heart disease 92–3,
        95
    dummy cigarettes 103
    during pregnancy 95
    health risks 92–4
    help to quit 102–4
    herbal cigarettes 103
    how to give up 99–102
    and hypertension 152
    and mortality 93
    national figures for 96–7
    nicotine products 104
    non-nicotine deterrents 104
    passive smoking 62, 94–5
    pipes and cigars 98–9
    reasons for giving up 92–4, 99
    self-help groups 103
    and stress 97–8
    and vitamin deficiency 75
    and weight worries 97
    withdrawal symptoms 100–1
    women on HRT 130

spastic colon 191
sprains 19, 190
squash 54, 60
stair-climbers 51
stamina 15
step aerobics 54–5
stomach upsets 110
strains 19
strength 15–16
stress
    benefits of exercise 14
    coping with 8, 187–9
    definition 166
    environmental pressures 177
    fear of crime 182–3
    good time management 184–7
    habituation 168, 170
    individual responses to 177–8
    levels of 170
    life events and 172–4
    life stage and 175–7, 181
    life style and 174–5, 181
    optimum levels 165
    overstress 181–3
    pain and 171–2
    physical responses 167–8, 169
    and sexual problems 116, 134, 165
    smoking and 97–8
    social pressures 177
    sources of 172–80
    stress-related illnesses 165–6
    symptoms 170–1
    therapies and relaxation techniques
        189–99
    understress 180–1
    work and 179–80, 183–4
stretch classes 55
stretching exercises 28–35
strokes 14, 16, 17, 23, 66, 85, 93,
    150, 151, 157–8
sugar 69, 81
sunbathing 141–2
suppleness 15, 28
swimming 39, 55–6

table tennis 56–7
t'ai chi 197–8
tennis 57, 60
testicular cancer 143
testosterone 89, 114, 133

thrombosis 23
time management 184–7
tinnitus 110
tranquillisers 189
transient ischaemic attack (TIA)
    157–8
treadmills 51

ulcers 94, 190

vaginal dryness 122
varicose veins 27
vegans 75
vegetarians 75
visualisation techniques 198
vitamin supplements 74–5
vitamins 73–4, 140
voluntary work
    groups and organisations in need
        209, 210
    reasons for volunteering 208
    training opportunities 207
    University of the Third Age 210
    Voluntary Service Overseas
        209–10

walking 39, 49–50, 52–3
weight control
    alcohol and 105, 106
    and blood pressure 152
    body mass index (BMI) 88
    body shape and 89
    commercial slimming products 90

diets 89
ex-smokers 97
exercise and 14
fibre and 70
herbal slimming patches 90
obesity 14, 87–8, 190
testosterone patches 89
underweight 88
see also healthy eating
weight training 58–9, 61
weights 53, 59
women
    breast cancer 14, 129, 141, 142–3
    heart disease 125–6, 146–7
    menstrual cycle 119–21
    pregnancy 95, 116–18
    reproductive system 122
    sexual difficulties 115
    'superwoman syndrome' 180
    see also female menopause;
        hormone replacement therapy
        (HRT);
osteoporosis
work
    shift work 179
    stress and 179–80, 183–4
    'superwoman syndrome' 180
    workaholism 179

yoga 39, 59, 198–9

zinc 77, 79

CARING FOR PARENTS IN LATER LIFE

Taking responsibility for an elderly parent or parent-in-law can be quite a challenge, even for those who have hitherto enjoyed a close, loving relationship with their relative. *Caring for Parents in Later Life* offers advice on practical, financial and legal matters, and helps carers cope with all aspects of looking after an older relative.

Among the topics covered are:
- where the elderly person will live – own home, carer's home, sheltered accommodation or residential home
- practical aids and domestic adaptations that can help the infirm remain self-reliant longer
- legal considerations
- financial concerns
- how to help someone come to terms with the death of a spouse
- how to face up to the emotional strains and stresses
- symptoms of physical and mental deterioration to look out for in the elderly, and when to seek medical advice.

In addition, an invaluable 'help directory' lists addresses, telephone numbers, services and literature available to both carer and dependant.

Paperback   216 x 135mm   272 pages

Available from bookshops,
including the Which? shop at
359-361 Euston Road, London NW1,
and by post from
Consumers' Association, Dept TAZM,
Castlemead, Gascoyne Way, Hertford X, SG14 1LH.

Access/Visa card holders can phone FREE on
(0800) 252100 to place their order,
quoting Dept TAZM.

THE WHICH? GUIDE TO PENSIONS

Whether you are taking the first steps towards joining a pension scheme or are wondering how to boost your existing pension, this book will help you make the right pre-retirement decisions.

The ever-increasing range of pensions available – from different kinds of employer and state pension schemes to personal pension plans – makes it more important than ever to choose a scheme you can trust and avoid potentially expensive mistakes.

The Which? Guide to Pensions contains reliable information on how to build up valuable funds for when you retire and offers advice on pension safety, women and pensions, and alternatives to pensions.

Throughout, case histories and charts help to elucidate this notoriously bewildering subject, and a glossary of pensionspeak provides instant clarification of the jargon.

Paperback   216 x 135mm   252 pages

Available from bookshops,
including the Which? shop at
359-361 Euston Road, London NW1,
and by post from
Consumers' Association, Dept TAZM,
Castlemead, Gascoyne Way, Hertford X, SG14 1LH.

Access/Visa card holders can phone FREE on
(0800) 252100 to place their order,
quoting Dept TAZM.

Other books from Consumers' Association

Understanding Headaches and Migraines – A practical guide to avoiding and coping with all forms of headache

Understanding HRT and the Menopause – Managing 'the change' with or without hormone replacement therapy

Understanding Stress – The causes and symptoms, and the most effective methods of stress management

Understanding Back Trouble – How to prevent, treat and cope with back trouble

Preventing Heart Disease – Understanding and taking care of your heart

The Which? Guide to Men's Health – The essential health and fitness manual for men and those who care about them

Which? Medicine – The essential consumer guide to over 1,500 medicines in common use

All are available from bookshops, including the Which? shop at 359-361 Euston Road, London NW1 (telephone: 071-830 7640); and by post from Consumers' Association, Castlemead, Gascoyne Way, Hertford X, SG14 1LH

Access/Visa cardholders can phone FREE on (0300) 252100 to place their order

---

Free trial subscription to *Which? way to Health*

Whether you want positive advice on staying fit, a healthy diet or detecting health problems at an early stage, *Which? way to Health* magazine is for you. Published every two months, it gives you the results of tests on health products, and practical advice to help you take control of your own health and lead a life style that will cut down health risks and keep stress levels in check.

Written in a clear, uncomplicated way, *Which? way to Health* gives you the plain facts without scientific jargon or marketing hype. It is truly independent: it takes no advertising, so it can tell you the things you want to know, not what advertisers want you to know. For details of our *free* trial subscription offer, write to Dept. E6, Consumers' Association, FREEPOST, Hertford X, SG14 1YB.